MEDICAL CARE
FOR THE AGED

MEDICAL CARE FOR THE AGED

From Social Problem to Federal Program

Henry P. Brehm
Rodney M. Coe

PRAEGER

PRAEGER SPECIAL STUDIES • PRAEGER SCIENTIFIC

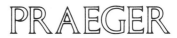

Library of Congress Cataloging in Publication Data

Brehm, Henry P
    Medical care for the aged.

    Bibliography: p.
    Includes index.
    1. Aged--Medical care--United States. 2. Aged--
Care and hygiene--United States. 3. Medicare.
4. Aged--Government policy--United States. I. Coe,
Rodney M., joint author. II. Title. [DNLM: 1. Health
insurance for aged and disabled, Title 18. 2. Delivery
of health care--In old age--United States. WT30 B834m]
RA413.7.A4B73   362.1'0880565   80-21026
ISBN 0-03-046306-8

Published in 1980 by Praeger Publishers
CBS Educational and Professional Publishing
A Division of CBS, Inc.
521 Fifth Avenue, New York, New York 10017 U.S.A.

© 1980 by Praeger Publishers

0123456789   145   987654321

Printed in the United States of America

**To
Molly and Elaine**

PREFACE

The authors of this book, in cooperation with other investigators, have used a particular analytic model in reviewing public policy relative to a series of social insurance and social welfare issues. The issues include meeting the economic needs of the disabled and widowed through Social Security and financing the medical care needs of the aged under Medicare.

The present volume discusses in detail the broader issues involved in meeting the medical care needs of the aged. It is one of a set of books that deal with the above-mentioned issues and attempt to address each separately using the same framework. These books assess the consistency of focus in the conception and identification of a social problem, formulation of a policy, and development and implementation of an action program. These books review the results of three Social Security Administration-funded studies with social policy implications. Each study is concerned with a different population category defined as in need of governmental action to ameliorate the impact of a social problem. In each case, a general policy for solving the problem has been translated into a legislated program. However, there is not necessarily an adequate fit between a general policy and the program designed to fulfill that general policy, nor does the policy necessarily indicate an accurate understanding and assessment of the underlying social problem.

In each of the three cases, two primary issues of policy analysis are considered: first, whether the general policy, conceptualized explicitly or implicitly for dealing with a specific social problem, is consonant with the parameters of the problem; and second, whether there is a fit between the policy and the social program—that is, whether the formally instituted program accomplishes the generally stated objectives in dealing with the underlying social problem. The first issue concerns both an adequate conception of the nature and root causes of that problem and an accurate assessment of its scope and dimensions. The second includes evaluation of government action involving implementing procedures and administrative rules established by the responsible agency.

Inconsistency or mismatch within these areas of concern may result in failure of a social program independently of the level of funding or the operating efficiency of program administration. No attempt is made here to assess program administration efficiency, per se. This study is oriented

Portions of this presentation are based on *Impact of Medicare in Selected Communities*, by Rodney M. Coe, Warren E. Peterson, Jack Sigler, Mary Stroker, and Julie Edgerton. Final Report SSA Contract No. 71-3400, April 1973.

toward the formulation and implementation of policy and the outcome of the program.

The possible reasons for mismatch at the level of the definition of the problem embodied in the general policy or at the level of the legislated program designed to accomplish the goals of the policy are examined in detail. Some possible reasons for a mismatch include: (1) a lack of appropriate data on the nature or dimensions of the problem or on what actions might affect it and how; (2) the irresolution of opposing philosophies on approaches to be taken toward or responsibilities for social problems; and (3) political compromise negotiated between or for vested interest groups with varying degrees of power.

The analytic framework of problem, policy, and program is used in dealing with the three social problem areas mentioned: the economic needs of the widowed, the economic needs of the disabled, and the medical care needs of the aged. The policies for dealing with these social problems on which we are focusing our attention are public income maintenance for the widowed and the disabled, and the financing of medical care for the aged. The three specific programs under consideration are Social Security Survivors Insurance and Disability Insurance, and Health Insurance for the Aged (Medicare).

The contention is that some of the deficiencies observed in program outcomes in the three problem areas may be based on a mismatch at either or both of the levels discussed. If there is such a mismatch, the result of the program might be contrary to the intent of the general policy approach designed to deal with the social problem.

If this happens and the problem is not properly identified, proposed solutions may be inappropriate. As an example, if data indicate a given program appropriately matches the policy formulated and that the difficulty in a lack of program "success" is that the policy itself does not reflect a clear understanding of the underlying social problem, then strengthening administration of the program will not be effective. Similarly, supplying additional funds for program implementation, or making minor changes in the legislative structure of the program or its implementing procedures and administrative regulations will not be effective in improving outcomes. It would be necessary to review at the appropriate level what a new policy should be, and to redesign the legislated program and its implementation to deal with the underlying social problem as redefined or reassessed.

METHODS OF PROCEDURE

The three studies that provide the major inputs for these individual volumes perform analyses using data from three separate and distinct methodological approaches. The analytic model is addressed to independent although potentially overlapping areas of social problems.

The study on medical care for the aged, discussed in detail in this volume, uses data collected from individuals in a representative sample of households and community medical facilities in five midwestern communities. The analysis reported here relates primarily to data from a major midwestern metropolitan area. Comparable cross-sectional data were collected for three separate times: the period prior to the implementation of Medicare; two years after the implementation of Medicare; and again two years later.

One conclusion drawn is that the policy of providing the aged with greater access to medical care through relief from the pressures of financing this care fit only one aspect of the underlying social problem, that of the need among the aged for assistance in financing care under circumstances of decreased financial means. Other important dimensions of the problem, such as availability of services, were not included in the policy statement. Thus, the program does not alter the system of providers for delivering medical care to the American population in general and the aged in particular. These issues, and their implications for health care policy and program, will be considered specifically in the chapters that follow.

Disability

For the study on disability, the analysis was based on data from the 1970 U.S. Census of Population, on Social Security Disability Insurance (SSDI) program data on application for and award of benefits, and on State Disability Determination Services characteristics. Analysis was done of differences among states in the rates of self-defined disability and application for and award of benefits under the Social Security Disability Insurance program, as these related to state economic and social conditions. Analysis was done of the administrative characteristics of state DDSs as these related to the rates of award.

The companion volume *Disability* reviews the background and developmental history of the present legislation authorizing the Social Security Disability Insurance program and describes the social problem towards which the underlying policy was aimed. The findings indicate the policy clearly was aimed at a medical conception of the problem of disability. However, evidence exists to indicate that the self-definition of disability in the population and, hence, the tendency to apply for disability benefits are based in large measure on the capacity of individuals actually to get and hold jobs. It appears that the number of people who define themselves as disabled and, therefore, take action based on that definition may be highly related to the social and economic circumstances of the state in which they live, rather than principally to the specific health problem with which they may individually be affected.

The evidence indicated that the rate of award of benefits to the insured population is based on the rate of applications. Similar evidence indicated that the award of benefits is also related to aspects of the separate state-by-state administration of the disability determination process. There are two possible interpretations for these data. One would suggest the possibility that more weight is given in the determination process to the underlying social and economic characteristics of the state than was intended under the legislated program or its implementing regulations. In this situation, the state-administered disability determination process is seen as responsive to pressures within the state.

The second interpretation would suggest that under given negative economic characteristics, that is, factors that indicate difficulty in getting and holding a job in the state, more people with legitimate health or injury characteristics may apply for benefits. Since these people can meet the medical impairment standards for disability, they will be awarded benefits independent of any particular emphasis placed on social and economic factors. In this situation, the point at issue is not whether these people meet the standards, but whether their basis for applying for benefits is their health as a factor affecting their ability to engage in substantial gainful activity, or the economic situation that restricts the ability to gain a position in substantial gainful activity. Since the population with one or more chronic diseases by far exceeds the number who report themselves as disabled, there may be a vast reservoir of people who could define themselves as disabled if they found themselves in a restricted job market that, therefore, promoted and reinforced their definitions of themselves as disabled as a result of their impairments.

By focusing on listings of medical impairments that might serve as a general standard of disability for the average worker on the average job, the disability insurance program created a structure in which disability is viewed in terms of its underlying medical cause rather than as a limitation of function that inhibits substantial gainful activity and that may have resulted from a medically definable impairment. The result of the program's focus on medical impairment as the equivalent of disability is that it is subject to a great deal of pressure in the form of applications based on economic circumstances.

The massive growth of the SSDI program in the last few years may relate only in part to the data presented here. However, there does appear to be a misfit between the underlying social problem, that is, the population basis for self-definition of disability and application for benefits, and the definitions and goals expressed in the policy for dealing with the problem of disability, as well as between the policy and the actual program as implemented.

Widowhood

For the study of widowhood, there was a household survey of current and recent past beneficiaries, with a small sampling of widows who had received only a lump sum burial benefit. The interview asked about the various support systems available to and used by the widow for her economic, social, and emotional support. The companion volume *Widowhood* is on the economic support of the widow and its relationship to her current life-cycle situation.

In the area of benefits for the widowed population, the policy formulated to deal with the social problem seems not to have recognized the full extent of two aspects of the problem of widowhood. One is that widows who either are caring for minor children, or are themselves of relatively advanced age, are not the only widows in need of help or assistance. Also, the possibility that the present generation of widows has unique characteristics unlike those of generations of widows to follow has not been taken into specific consideration in the formulation of a policy and implementation of a program. The present generation of widows has a higher percentage of women who were either born outside the United States, or were married to men born outside the United States, than is anticipated in future generations of widows. As a result, these widows and their husbands often received only minimal education. Many of these women did not work under the social security system themselves and had husbands who earned relatively low levels of benefits under the system. The enactment of a program to care for the needs of a generation of widows including many women such as those just described would not necessarily be the same type of program appropriate for a generation of widows more of whom were born in the United States, received higher levels of education, and married men who had more education than their predecessors. The husbands of such women had better jobs and were entitled to higher retirement benefits, and their widows were entitled to higher benefits as survivors. Also, these widows were more likely to work under the system and earn benefits in their own right.

The size of the population of women in the U.S. who were widows at approximately the time of the study is indicated by reference to the 1970 census. The highest percentage of beneficiary widows are 60 years of age and over, the age at which they can receive benefits based on age. The women in the study who are younger than 60 are either current mothers of minor children and are receiving benefits based on the age of their children; ex-beneficiaries whose children are too old to permit the payment of benefits based on the care of the husband's dependent children, or who have remarried; or women who received only lump sum burial benefits.

An omission in the formal program as it relates to the general policy of caring for widows is any form of transitional coverage or other assistance for the widow who is not old enough herself to receive benefits based on age but whose youngest child has reached majority. This group is totally omitted from the social security program despite the existence of a social problem. For these women there is no SSA program to help them re-enter the job market or otherwise reorganize their lives.

It is understandable that no direct benefit would be paid to a widow in her young fifties who was not disabled. However, many women in that age group have left the job market, and while many are potentially capable of re-entry not all are currently equipped to do so. By concentrating primarily on the needs of the young widow with minor children, many of whom could also be helped to re-enter the job market and may also soon reach the transitional period, and the needs of the older widow who represents a unique generation that may be passing out of existence, we have ignored the needs of the widow in between, whom for practical purposes we have defined as a nonwidow.

This is the thrust of this set of books. It is our hope they will contribute to the literature on policy formulation and program planning as related to the handling of social problems, and also to a better understanding of the issues in each of the specific areas of concern.

CONTENTS

LIST OF TABLES

1
HEALTH: DEFINING
THE PROBLEM,
SETTING POLICY,
DESIGNING A PROGRAM

INTRODUCTION

The major purpose of this book is to review Medicare from the analytic perspective of the match between the social problem presented by a lack of adequate health care for the aged, the formulated policy and the implemented program to resolve the problem, and the implications of this match for effectiveness in dealing with the underlying problem. Reviewing public programs to deal with the health care needs of the aged requires a broad perspective that places this social policy area within a more general framework of both health and social welfare issues in the United States. To provide a review of the context in which the problem was defined, and in which the policy and program were framed, we will discuss briefly some general considerations in society's value orientation and approach to health and social welfare issues.

First, however, let us set forth the definitions we use for the terms problem, policy, and program and provide some background on the importance of problem definition for effective public policy. We define "problem" as a situation or condition that negatively affects a significant portion of the population and that requires collective action for solution. Circumstances that do not conform to social expectations or that impede social performance would meet this definition (Ryan, 1976). The aged, because of increased frequency and severity of disease, often have restrictions in their capacity for social performance. However, this situation interacts with other circumstances faced by the aged, such as limited incomes, with the result that the problem can be defined and approached from several perspectives.

"Policy," as we use the term, is a set of general statements of goals and objectives embodied implicitly or explicitly in legislation to address the problem. Policy for dealing with a problem is established when society, through its agents, assumes a degree of responsibility for relief of the problem as defined in the policy and adopts a course of action.

The course of action adopted is formalized as the "program," which, in our use of the word, is the action aspect of policy. It is a set of specific benefits or services provided and the procedures, eligibility requirements, and so on designed for administrative management.

The Focus on Problem Definition

A series of social value judgements is involved in how a problem is defined and in deciding upon a policy direction to deal with it. Social problems can be viewed from more than one perspective, depending upon the vantage point of the viewer, the availability of information about the overall situation, and the factors related to both occurrence and potential resolution of the problem, including other, competing social values of the society. The problem underlying social policy almost always has alternative definitions, and solutions to the problem may be approached in various ways.

Additionally, there are long-term trends in social value structures that characterize society and its approach to social problems. Social values are not static. Hence, the approach to and definition of a social problem may not necessarily be consistent throughout society at any given point in time, nor does it always move only in one direction for trends over time.

There are, as a result, competing philosophies that may require compromises between advocates of different positions and modifications in a proposed approach before social policy to deal with a problem is worked out and established in a program. The program may then change over a period of years in an incremental movement of social policy (Braybrooke and Lindholm, 1963). The program may also change based on the introduction of modifications presumably designed to improve or simplify administration, for efficiency or equity. These may be intended as technical modifications not designed to introduce a change in policy, but they can result in more far-reaching effects than anticipated.

The dominant value system of society can result in traditional responses to identification and definition of a problem by those occupying positions of leadership. The interweaving of traditional concepts of problems and their solutions into our social values may limit the range of creativity in seeking solutions.

This point is amply illustrated by Dexter in *Tyranny of Schooling*. His analysis, using the problem of education of the borderline mentally retarded and their relationship to the public school system as an example, indicates the potential for redefining a problem using another approach.

The United States has an established tradition of providing a basic education to all children. Our value system supports schooling as an essential ingredient in the formula for success in adult life, for both employment and general citizenship. We include some measure of educational attainment as a prerequisite for employment even in positions where the connection between schooling and job performance requirements is at best tenuous. Under these circumstances, how do we deal with the problem defined as the inability of some children to perform adequately in absorbing a basic education?

Our value system is achievement-oriented, and we see education as the cornerstone of achievement. We attempt to instill the value of education as part of the schooling process for children who are not reached by our educational system because of cultural background or personal preference. What will happen to the child who rejects schooling? What will happen to society if this is allowed to occur too often? For children who have difficulty absorbing an education through no fault of their own, we tend to make schooling an ordeal. Our social values say they must attend school and must learn. The problem and the solution are viewed in traditional, relatively inflexible ways.

Dexter presents a strong rationale for the possibility of redefining the problem created by the poor school performance of the borderline mentally retarded. He points out that members of this select group among the retarded run into trouble with society primarily in their encounter with the formal education system. The data he presents indicate that they are not a social problem because of higher crime rates, needs for institutionalization, or an inability to be trained for job levels that afford them the potential for self-support. They cannot function properly in standard public schools, and this creates difficulties for them, as well as for the conventional school system.

Dexter suggests that the problem may have been framed inaccurately. Perhaps the problem is not so much borderline mental retardation as it is universal compulsory childhood education. Compulsory education is thoroughly ingrained in our child-rearing practices, our legal structure, and our educational standards for employment. To consider it the problem rather than mental retardation runs contrary to all our preconceptions and social values. However, it provides an excellent message. We accept certain definitions of social problems because we have been conditioned by our social value system to view them that way. Dexter does not indicate he espouses this definition of the problem, but merely cites this approach to mental retardation and compulsory education as an alternative possibility. We need not accept this approach to accept the point that our conceptions of social problems are socially determined. Examining alternative definitions of a social problem provides a broader framework within which to establish policy to deal with it.

With respect to the issue of health, disease is usually defined in our society as a medically determinable mental or physical condition that may threaten the life or impair the functioning of the affected individual. There is a reasonable consensus on how and why diseases generally affect people and what the problem is. Criteria for identification of "who," "when," and "where" are available and are applied with minimal disagreement about whose standards should be applied. However, there are exceptions to agreement in the definition of specific conditions as disease. Alcoholism and drug addiction sometimes also are viewed moralistically and treated as sin or crime with or without the identification of a specific victim. The approaches to dealing with them from this view are often punitive or involve atonement and self-control efforts.

Even when it is agreed that a particular condition is a disease, opinion differs on whether the nature of the problem should be conceptualized individually or collectively. Do we put major emphasis on helping the sick, on protecting the well, or on trying to balance both approaches even if it means less than a full effort in either direction? Sometimes these objectives are compatible; sometimes they are contradictory. Isolating plague victims protects the rest of society; establishing care facilities is an attempt to help the victim, but may increase the risks that the disease will spread. Often, resources may be too limited to accomplish both objectives.

For diseases that are not epidemic and immediately life-threatening, do we focus on prevention or cure? Do we deal with the environmental aspects of disease occurrence and spread, with the individual aspects, or with both, by distributing limited total resources in two directions? Do we attempt to obtain additional resources not initially devoted to health concerns to mount an effective effort in both directions? Do we define the problem relative to the environmental causes of disease or relative to the individual's ability to avoid disease? Is disease a problem because of its physical effects or because of its social or financial results? As for medical care itself, do we consider technical quality, equal access, coordination of resources, assistance for cost, or some other aspect? How we view the problem has implications for how we approach it, particularly since there are always limitations on society's resources, and a focus on one view of a problem may limit the ability to deal with it from another, incompatible perspective.

There is general agreement on the definition of some diseases as social problems in that they result from environmental risks that are either "natural," "uncontrollable" events or based on collective or individual human acts. However, there are different conceptions of the nature of the problem, which require different approaches for dealing with it. Ryan (1976) and Crawford (1977) have both reviewed the issue of holding the individual responsible for his or her own health status. The concern they express over this view is not that it relates to providing health improvement programs to promote public awareness of individual actions that decrease the risks of illness or foster good health. The concern is that efforts to hold the individual responsible for his or her health status may be seen as an alternative to providing health services. Health care is increasingly expensive and an economic burden on the population in general, including those who do attempt to adjust their life styles to protect their health. Blaming illness on the individual might provide a rationale for a reduced effort by society to resolve social problems related to lack of access to and affordability of health services.

The chapters that follow will review conceptions of the problem of the health of the aged and how this problem was and might have been defined in formulating the policy that gave rise to the Medicare program. We will then attempt to assess experience under the program from the perspective of the problem it was designed to deal with, using the analytic approach of the match among the original problem, the policy, and the program.

THE CONTEXT OF SOCIAL VALUES

It is not possible to divorce the approaches and mechanisms used in programs addressed to the health needs of the aged from the overall societal view of health and health care, and public responsibility for dealing with these concerns. Similarly, the social value orientation toward responsibility for public provision of specific services, paying for certain private services, and directly providing general income maintenance affects how the health needs of the aged will be met.

Defining the problem of the health of the aged, formulating a policy to deal with the problem, and developing a program to carry out the policy occurred against the background of social values concerning health and social welfare. Medicare resulted from a merging of the social values regarding these two areas of concern.

The Context of Social Values in Health and Health Care

The World Health Organization defines health as a state of "complete physical, mental, and social well-being and not merely the absence of disease" (Longest, 1979, p. 341). A series of factors is involved in the health of individuals, including human biology, environmental conditions, and lifestyle (behavioral) considerations. Health services are activities intended to help the individual maintain or improve health. As Longest suggests, these can be divided into three basic types: public health services conducted on a community basis; environmental health services, which often overlap public health services, but are involved specifically with efforts to reduce disease contagion through environmental control; and personal health services for individuals, directed at health promotion, illness prevention, diagnosis, treatment, and rehabilitation. The health care system that provides these health services is only one of the factors affecting the health status of the population. However, estimates of current federal health expenditures suggest that approximately $9 out of every $10 spent on determinants of health status are spent on the health care system. The remainder is used for environmental, biological, and behavioral determinants. At the same time, the health care system is seen mostly as a source of intervention after disease has become manifest. As a result it is very limited in its impact on the health of the population. It is, in this sense, a vital line of defense for the health of the population because preventive measures relative to environmental, biological, and behavioral determinants have been insufficient or ineffective (Longest, 1979).

The practicing physician is the professional controlling the use of personal health services. The health care obtained by individuals has been a matter of direct dealings between the patient and the physician as prime provider. While limitations have been set on who may practice medicine, government policy in the United States to date has avoided directly interfering in the doctor-patient relationship, exercising control over the practice of medicine or how medical care is provided, or limiting the free choice of physician by the patient. As we shall see later, these were central principles specified in the Medicare authorizing legislation.

In attempting to understand the physician's position relative to society and his individual patients, it should be recognized that "at no time in history did he have anything like a complete monopoly over healing services, informal or formal." Patients cannot be prevented from treating themselves or from seeking nonprofessional help from friends or relatives. "A complete formal monopoly has never been granted medicine by the state. In modern times legal exceptions to the monopoly are few but exist nonetheless. . . . In past times, exceptions to monopoly were the rule" (Freidson, 1972, p. 17).

The title "doctor" conferred by a university was the first stable indicator by which a respectable healer could be distinguished from other practitioners. The development of medical schools within universities and of physician guilds facilitated formal regulation of occupations related to health by giving specific public identity to the physician. Early examples of this date back to the twelfth and thirteenth centuries. However, these did not establish a monopoly over healing for the physician because they could not create widespread public confidence in and use of physician services (Freidson, 1972).

The early doctors of this country were at considerable distance from the nearest medical professor and source of drugs in the Old World. Efforts to establish domestic medical institutions had just started when the American Revolution began. These doctors worked to cure the sick under the harsh conditions of a newly developing nation, often without any formal training (Flexner, 1969).

By the nineteenth century, no single group of healers had obtained a real, as contrasted to formally sponsored, monopoly over healing services. Public confidence was lacking and the physician was not accorded great authority as a healer. There was a variety of healing movements and approaches in the United States. The conditions of an expanding frontier and a spirit of egalitarianism made it impossible to impose or enforce restrictions on who might practice healing. This lack of clear restrictions played a part in preventing the scientific advances of the nineteenth century from being well assimilated or conveyed to the public (Freidson, 1972).

The relationship between disease and the social and economic conditions in which people live had been systematically expressed as early as the latter part of the eighteenth century. The relationship between disease and the environment was further elaborated upon in the mid-nineteenth century. While there were recommendations for social action, this early work cannot be said to have had an immediate effect on public policy. It did introduce a new idea for the time—that many deaths are preventable (Gordon et al., 1968).

The bacteriological breakthrough, which led to the discovery in the latter part of the nineteenth century of the specific causes for specific diseases, joined the correct conclusion about the relationship of disease and the environment to the correct theory. This led to a series of successes in dealing with common infectious diseases. It also caused the bulk of research effort to be directed toward the disease agent and away from the host and the social and physical environment.

It was not until after 1915 that the relationships between death and disease rates and economic level were established with some precision. "It was not until the nature of medical practice had evolved to something akin to the structure we know today that concern arose over the effective use of the health apparatus that had been developing for a century" (Gordon et al., 1968, p. 11). In the interim, over 4,000 general hospitals were built (from 1875 to 1910) and the basis of medical education was revolutionized (from 1910 to 1920) (Gordon et al., 1968).

It was not until the early twentieth century that physician licensing was widely established in this country. This licensure was based on uniform standards for medical education. With the combination of political consolidation of the United States and a sound technical basis for physician training, licensure laws could be enforced and the physician could gain the confidence of the public. The result was that the medical profession could establish the justice of its claim to privilege in practicing healing and obtain "control over the practice of healing that has never before been enjoyed by medicine" (Freidson, 1972, p. 21).

To summarize this discussion of the context of social values in health and health care within which the problem of the health of the aged was defned and the policy and program underlying Medicare were formed, it is apparent that efforts to deal directly with the health of the population had not particularly been in evidence in terms of governmental action. Those efforts that had been undertaken were primarily directed toward public health and environmental health services. Before Medicare and Medicaid, which, as we will discuss, relate to financing and not direct provision or standards for care, government involvement in personal health services for the population as a whole basically centered on licensure and training standards for medical care practitioners.

In effect, the health of the general population historically has been defined primarily as an individual responsibility and not as a public responsibility. In the past, for the bulk of the population direct governmental policy on health basically extended only to providing an environment as safe as possible from infectious diseases and protecting the rest of society from serious communicable diseases by isolating the sick. Individuals were expected to exercise caution in exposing themselves to disease and to make their own arrangements for seeking care when they did fall prey to sickness. Even in times of major epidemics, governmental attempts to intervene in the situation placed emphasis on protecting the healthy members of society from the spread of disease, not on treating the individual. In more recent concerns for "blaming the victim" (Ryan, 1976), the most significant issue is probably not that there is any break with the past in the focus on individual responsibility for maintaining personal health, but that there is an increased awareness of environmental factors under public control that may influence health risks. Additionally, there are now potentially effective care mechanisms available and public resources that can be devoted to treating individuals. That is, we can increasingly do something about health problems, although an expenditure of scarce and expensive resources is required.

However, the health of Americans and the delivery of health care services to the population has been a continuing concern of health professionals, politicians, and consumers. Individual physicians have been involved in delivering medical care services to Americans since well before there was an "American" government. Military medicine, though poorly supplied and organized, was practiced in support of the troops fighting in the American Revolution. As far back as 1798, there existed the forerunner of the United States Public Health Service, with its historical mission of protecting the health of the population through control of the spread of contagious diseases and direct medical care of specified categories of persons, that is, American Indians, merchant marines, coast guardsmen, and others for whom the federal government takes responsibility. There is a long record of public health activity aimed at protecting the health of the population through environmental controls such as the inspection and safeguarding of clean water and food supplies and the regulation of sanitary conditions. But with the exception of the special categories listed above and the care available to those in the military, to their dependents, and to veterans, government action at the time Medicare was considered had not traditionally been oriented toward attempts to provide direct care. Federal and state government units directly operated or supported screening for specific diseases, maternal and child health clinics, treatment facilities for tuberculosis, and special care programs. Responsibility had not been taken for providing directly for the general medical care needs of major segments of the civilian population, or for exercising control over the organization or financing of such care. These issues were left in the hands of the medical profession, local providers, and insurers. Some limited governmental arrangements were available to provide care for indigents, and local governments in some locations operated city and county hospitals. In no sense did these latter efforts satisfy the needs for care even of the most indigent population.

The Context of Social Values in Social Welfare

As we will see in Chapter 3, the first efforts in this country to provide a government-sponsored national program of health insurance predate the establishment of our basic social welfare and social insurance programs. However, the eventual approval of a program of health insurance covering only the aged portion of the population followed by three decades the passage of the original version of the Social Security Act. In the interim, a health insurance industry had grown much beyond the original modest efforts to pool risks as a way of assuring that medical care bills would be paid. The scope and form of the industry and the health insurance plans offered were affected by developments during World War II. Public programs of health care financing were developed from the perspective of population coverage and eligibility determination and modeled after the basic income maintenance approaches seen in the Social Security Act. The approach to services covered and reimbursement was modeled after that of nongovernmental third-party payment health insurance plans. The impact of Blue Cross-Blue Shield and other health insurance plans on the development of Medicare will be discussed in Chapter 3. The relationship between public programs of income maintenance in general and medical care benefits in particular are of concern here.

Public Services and Income Maintenance

A variety of services for the public is provided directly by government at some level. Police and fire protection, street lighting, road building and maintenance, trash removal, and education are examples of services available to all citizens and commonly financed through general or special-purpose taxes. As discussed earlier, an array of public health services is usually provided on this basis. Direct medical care services, however, are usually excluded, except for special population groups.

In the case of certain other services not directly provided by a government unit, government may provide specific payment or reimbursement for a service or subsidize a service with the intent of assuring public availability of the service, usually free of charge or at reduced cost. Medical care services paid for under Medicare or Medicaid fall into this category. The financing for such services may come from general or special taxes. There may be some restrictions on eligibility for receipt of these services. Those eligibility criteria that do exist may relate to economic circumstances, among other considerations. When the economic circumstances of the potential service recipients are a consideration, the program is conceptually related to the more general approach of income maintenance. Public income maintenance directly provides individuals and families with money with which to buy goods and services. While assumptions are made about needed levels of income or amount of prior earnings to be replaced, the use of these funds is basically left to the discretion of the recipient.

The two general categories of public income maintenance are universal and income or means tested programs. Universal programs are available for all members of society who meet prescribed eligibility criteria not specifically tied to economic circumstances. However, these criteria may identify groups of persons presumed categorically to require financial assistance, such as the disabled or those of retirement age. Means or income tested programs have specific financial status requirements in addition to any other eligibility criteria.

These two approaches to income maintenance were incorporated into separate aspects of the original Social Security Act of 1935. The Old Age Benefits program, which in time became Old-Age, Survivors, and Disability Insurance (OASDI), reflected the universal approach of social insurance. Survivors insurance was added in 1939, and disability insurance in 1956. The assistance programs of Aid to Dependent Children (later expanded to Aid to Families with Dependent Children and Aid to Families with Dependent Children with an Unemployed Parent (AFDC and AFDC-U), Aid to the Blind (AB), and Old Age Assistance (OAA) reflected the means or income tested approach of public welfare.

In 1965, the financing of medical care services under the Health Insurance for the Aged (Medicare) program was added as part of the social insurance approach. The Medicaid program, instituted at the same time as Medicare, followed the public welfare approach.

The Medicare program, which is our concern in this book, does not exist in isolation. It is part of the overall system of old-age, survivors, disability, and health insurance* that makes up the social security program of the United States. We need to review the developmental history of social security in the United States because of the implications this has for the approach taken toward government involvement in meeting the medical care needs of the aged under Medicare.

A BACKGROUND TO THE SOCIAL SECURITY ACT OF 1935

The 1920s reflected a period in American history when there was general contentment and expectation of economic prosperity. Accordingly, no overwhelming need was felt for drastic change in attitudes about who should get aid, nor was there significant support for provision by the national government of extensive programs of social welfare.

The sense of prosperity of the 1920s seemed to reduce the intensity of the confrontation between opposing views of government. Many were concerned that governmental tinkering would serve only to curb what seemed to be ever increasing and everlasting economic opportunities in this country. However, the depression of the 1930s had an impact upon such views.

The change in attitude was inevitable, given the fact that by 1933 over 25 percent of the civilian labor force was unemployed and approximately 40 percent of the population in some of the states was on relief (Clarke, 1957). While some continued to argue in favor of limited governmental intervention, the magnitude of the economic crisis resulted in the development of New Deal liberalism. Those who favored this approach maintained that the capitalist system could be salvaged only by recognizing that the situation called for more extensive central government involvement.

Social welfare programs in the U.S. formed a "patchwork of programs and assumptions" when the Social Security Act of 1935 was passed. There was "no unified social-welfare tradition" upon which to base this legislation (Stevens and Stevens, 1974). The possibility had been accepted that at least those who were obviously innocent victims of situations over which they had no control deserved somewhat better care. As a result, programs of "outdoor" relief were developed by the states to aid the aged poor, the blind, and dependent children. By the end of 1934, 28 states had passed old-age assistance programs that, in effect, removed the aged poor from almshouses. By 1935, 27 states provided payments for the blind. State programs for child

---

*The Department of Health, Education, and Welfare was reorganized in 1977, with responsibility for the administration of the Medicare program being transferred to the Health Care Financing Administration. However, eligibility for Medicare is still based on social security coverage and the program is financed using Social Security trust fund monies.

relief focused on providing aid to needy widows with dependent children. By 1934, all but 3 states provided such aid.

The depression of the 1930s caused even those of a more conservative orientation to acknowledge that the economic crisis had produced people in need despite their industry and exercise of individual initiative. Accordingly, there was general agreement that the national government should provide benefits as long as they were financed by an earmarked payroll tax. Even those committed to individualism could take comfort in this approach, because of its similarity to private insurance, in which people pay premiums in anticipation of a possible future need. Thus, "social insurance" reaffirmed the virtues of individual industry and initiative.

A stronger view was taken in some quarters of the kind of public welfare programs necessary in view of the economic crisis. In effect, the New Deal planners called for a broader assumption of governmental responsibility for public welfare, one in which general revenues would be used to support indigent people. Their position is implicit in the development of public assistance programs.

Social Insurance and the Social Security Act

The Social Security Act of 1935 was the product of a variety of pressures. The initial legislation and the program it established would be almost unrecognizable as anything more than the historic predecessor of today's act and program. But it established a precedent. For the first time in this country's history, the principle was established that it was legitimate through government effort to insure individual workers against the risks of loss of earning capacity in old age. The Great Depression both increased the pressures from various quarters for income guarantees and affirmed the fact that willing workers could find it impossible to obtain or hold jobs through no fault of their own.

It should not be assumed that the Social Security program of old-age insurance was instituted solely because of compassion for the welfare and the problems of older workers. The general economic situation was a major concern. It was apparent something would have to be done to prevent the economic dislocation of segments of the population in the future. The depression of the early 1930s forced a reassessment of our efforts to deal with the economy and its impact on people's lives. "The real roots of the Social Security Act were in the great depression. . . . Nothing else would have bumped the American people into a social security system except something so shocking, so terrifying, as that depression" (Perkins, 1962).

By the end of the first year of the Roosevelt administration, the various emergency measures the new president had set into motion to stimulate business recovery, stabilize the banking system, and relieve the plight of the unemployed were beginning to have an effect (Brown, 1972). The situation of economic collapse the president had faced at his inauguration in 1933 called for dramatic action to deal with the immediate effects of the depression: people had to be put back to work; business had to be stimulated; confidence in our economic system had to be restored. By early 1934, it was possible to think in terms of programs for the prevention of poverty and economic insecurity.

By this time the economic insecurity of the aged was becoming a major theme. The most popular of the movements for a radical mechanism to deal with this problem of the aged was the one backing the Townsend Plan. Dr. Townsend had put forward a plan for a flat $200 a month to be paid to each person over age 65, with the requirement that the money be spent so that this would produce a business stimulus. This "impossible miracle" gained vigorous support from normally conservative older people who accepted an image of economic salvation because of their deepening anxiety (Brown, 1972).

As J. Douglas Brown, one of the people called upon to help produce the proposals for the prevention of economic insecurity, phrased it much later,

It is difficult, thirty-five years later, to understand the effectiveness of the Townsend movement in exerting pressure on Congress. The scheme of supporting a $200 monthly grant to all people over 65 out of the proceeds of a greatly stimulated business activity caused by their expenditures was an extreme and faulty oversimplification of the function of money in a complex economy. But the compelling appeal was emotional, not economic. At the appeal's height, the supporters of the plan sent millions of postcards to their representatives in Congress. The most effective piece was a simple card depicting two scenes. One showed a forlorn old couple trudging up a snowy road with their few belongings. Underneath was the title, "over the Hill to the Poorhouse." The other picture showed the same couple seated before a cheery fire, the old lady knitting and the old man smoking his pipe. Its title was "Comfort in Old Age." Across the bottom of the card was the clearcut message, "Vote for the Townsend Plan" (Brown, 1972).

The plan's proposed approach for dealing with the economic plight of the aged was not realistic and acceptable, but it did have appeal. Providing improved purchasing power for the aged by a guaranteed income presented some potential concrete advantages. On the surface, it seemed that the plan would appropriately stimulate business by putting money into circulation. If older workers did not need employment to assure their incomes, they would not provide as much of a source of competition for jobs for younger workers. The movement for the Townsend Plan's adoption had to be sidetracked by the development of a more appropriate and reasonable program for preventing economic insecurity in old age.

> The beginning of old-age insurance came about largely . . . by the crisis of the times, by the studies of some of the intellectuals and through the impact of the old-age predicament, and of the Townsend organizations on the politicians (Perkins, 1963).

The combination of an increasing population of older Americans and an urban, industrial life style made a national contributory social insurance program a necessity. The issue became both moral and economic. "Full production must be supported by full consumption, and indigent people in a modern economy create a financial vacuum that endangers the whole structure . . ." (Tyler, 1955, p. 11). The emphasis in the social insurance approach is on the prevention of need resulting from specific probable risks rather than on providing relief after the individual proves poverty. The latter is the approach in public welfare or assistance, where the effort is directed toward immediate relief of existing poverty. The Social Security Act of 1935 incorporated both concepts into one document, although in different pieces of the program.

Making the social insurance part of the program contributory established that the benefit would be paid as a right based on the individual's own efforts. Aside from ensuring that benefit levels would be higher, relating benefits to individual contributions also made the program seem more related to individuals' efforts to help themselves. (Sanders, 1973). From the start, the social insurance program of old-age benefits was seen as appropriately national in scope, compulsory, and contributory. In addition, contributions were shared equally by the employer and the insured employee, and benefits were provided as a matter of right (Brown, 1972). These are still the basic principles on which the Old-Age, Survivors, and Disability Insurance program and the Medicare program are based.

A major concern in the initial effort to develop such a national old-age insurance program was the question of whether the United States government had the authority under the Constitution to establish such a program. From the current perspective the basis for such concern may seem doubtful. But in 1934, there was little to suggest the Constitution provided the authority to impose such a system on the citizens of this country (Brown, 1972).

Ultimately, the issue was resolved by recourse to the taxing power of the United States government. The social insurance program established under the Social Security Act is an appropriation mechanism that details the conditions under which benefits will be paid and the basis for computing benefit amounts. The program is financed through monies collected under the Federal Insurance Contributions Act (FICA), which is part of the Internal Revenue Code. The constitutionality of the program as established was affirmed by the United States Supreme Court within a few years after its passage.

Overview of the Social Security Program

The basic structure of the Old-Age, Survivors, and Disability Insurance program is a tax-transfer system. Contributions from current workers in covered employment are put into specially designated trust funds. Benefits are paid out of these trust funds to presently eligible retired or disabled workers or the survivors of deceased workers. Except for Medicare, where the benefits are the same for all eligible persons, the benefits paid are based on a formula dependent upon the workers' prior earnings in employment covered under the system. Eligibility is determined by whether the required technical standards for retirement, disability, or survivors benefits have been met and whether the worker has worked the necessary amount of time, as measured in quarters of coverage, under the system. While current employment is considered in determining whether the individual is indeed retired or disabled, and while there are limits set on the amounts beneficiaries can earn without a reduction in benefit amount, the individual's general economic condition, or need, is not a factor in determining eligibility for or amount of benefits to be received.

The formula used in determining the amount of benefit to which the worker (or the worker's survivors) is entitled provides a higher rate of replacement of prior earnings for workers with low average indexed earnings* in covered employment. Additionally, there is a minimum benefit to which workers with low average indexed earnings are entitled. These program features are designed to provide a degree of income adequacy from Social Security benefits for the low-income population. Efforts to move the Social Security benefit structure in this direction have been balanced by a concern for equity in the return on workers' contributions to the social insurance program.

The amount of contributions by workers and employers is based on a tax rate and a maximum amount of earnings in covered employment subject to the Federal Insurance Contributions Act (FICA) tax. These have changed periodically since the inception of the program. The taxable maximum in effect during given time periods results in limits on the average monthly indexed earnings level used for the computation of benefits.

As originally passed in 1935, the program provided benefits only to retired workers. It was an individual protection program. The program changed dramatically in 1939 to a family protection program by including dependent benefits for the wife and young children of retired workers and survivor benefits for the widow, orphans, and dependent parents of insured deceased workers. This program change related benefits to probable need as

---

*The 1977 amendments to the Social Security Act provided that for each year 1950 and later a worker's earnings are indexed relative to the average worker's earnings in that year. This increases the value for benefit computation of earnings from earlier years when average wages were lower.

evidenced by the existence of dependents (Sanders, 1973). The system no longer guaranteed to pay a lump-sum refund to individuals who reached age 65 without qualifying for a pension or to pay their estate on death what was paid into the program as FICA taxes (Tyler, 1955). If a worker qualified for no benefit, none was paid to him or on his account. These contributions were absorbed and actuarily adjusted for in the computation of revenues needed to pay the scheduled benefits.

A maximum benefit is prescribed that can be paid on any individual worker's account independent of the total number of eligible recipients. This family maximum ranges from 1.5 to about 1.8 times the individual worker's benefit.

The Social Security Act has been amended periodically over the years since its original passage. Most earlier amendments increased the number of employees covered under the program, the level of benefits, and the revenues for financing these benefits. The fundamental policy approach of the program as contributory and wage-related has basically been accepted as a permanent fixture, although alternate mechanisms for providing additional revenues for the system have been and very likely will be considered in the future.

The social insurance program of Social Security functions as a limited replacement for the worker's wages lost because of retirement, disability, or death. The benefits paid provide a floor of income on which to build other retirement income. The same approach was carried into Medicare when it was adopted some three decades after the basic program was established. The individual recipients are obliged to pay part of their own medical care costs.

The debate over the years about whether society had an obligation to provide medical care benefits even for workers who at age 65 were in need of financial support to help pay medical bills occurred against this philosophical background of social insurance and social welfare. We will discuss the development and specifics of the program in greater detail later. However, the intensity of this debate can be seen in some of the Medicare program features to be reviewed. The program pays for medical care provided by private vendors with administration divided between the national government and insurance companies acting as intermediaries. The individual's share of his or her total cost of care used is reflected in the deductible, co-insurance, and program exclusions. These are paid for either through the direct use of the individual's own funds or by arranging for the use of other payment sources, including privately obtained and paid-for insurance or, for those who can satisfy the economic need criteria, Medicaid. The assumption under Medicaid is that the individual cannot afford the costs of medical care and that, without the program's intervention, financial constraints would constitute a major barrier to obtaining needed medical care services. The policy intent was to remove this barrier entirely for individuals unable to pay for needed medical care. For the Medicare population, the cost of care was apparently conceived of as a burden to be lightened as a mechanism to facilitate the use of needed medical care services.

Relationship of Problem, Policy, and Program in Health Care for the Aged

The underlying objective of any government social policy and the program developed to implement it should be to provide relief from the effects of the target problem for the population directly affected by it. The present analysis is concerned with the degree of consistency among the social problem presented by the health needs of the aged, the policy designed to deal with it, and the specifics of the program and its implementing procedures developed to carry out the policy. This analytic approach suggests effective social programming can be stymied by inappropriate problem definition, inadequate policy formulation, or inconsistent program specification and implementation.

How adequately a social problem is defined in formulating policy is a critical issue in the congruence among problem, policy, and program, and determines the potential for successful problem amelioration. In the case of Medicare, the problem was defined in terms of the need for financial assistance among the aged in meeting the costs of health care. This problem focus and the policy and program for dealing with it have their roots in the general social values toward health and health care and the social insurance approach that existed in this country. The policy and program dealt only with payment for medical services delivered under the existing arrangements and did not address other approaches to providing care for the aged. The program established an insurance mechanism for paying for care actually received that followed the basic outline of Social Security.

METHODOLOGY OF DATA DEVELOPMENT

Various approaches were utilized in assembling the material presented here. They are discussed briefly in this section under the following categories: (1) identification of the problem; (2) policy formulation and program development; and (3) model analysis.

Identification of the Problem

There are several ways in which the problem of the health of the aged can be approached; each relates to a different base of data. It is appropriate for us to consider the issue from several perspectives, since these various views of the problem entered into the policy and program considerations underlying Medicare.

The health of the aged provided the point of reference for deliberations on the need to offer programmatic assistance for their health problems. Data on this issue were available from the Health Interview Survey (HIS) conducted by the National Center for Health Statistics (NCHS) and from special studies on the relationship of age to the distribution, severity, and effects of disease.

The data of primary concern are those that reflect the health situation of the aged when the policy and program debates surrounding Medicare were taking place. Additionally, one of the ways in which the impact of the program can be assessed is through a review of periodic health status data for the aged population.

The use of morbidity and mortality data for this purpose involves several serious difficulties. First, for the population at large, morbidity surveys rely on interview data composed of self-reports of symptoms and recall of diagnoses specified by a physician. These are subject to error from a variety of sources, including problems of faulty memory and differing levels of sophistication, as well as the possible existence of conditions for which medical attention was never sought or that were not labeled or identified for the individual.

A second difficulty is the possibility that concern for the health status of the aged and recognition of the need to do something about their problems will be equated with the expectation that any program will show a measurable improvement in specific health status indicators. It is not always possible to do something about the situation in a way that will show positive results for the morbidity or mortality rates among the aged. The ultimate result of the aging process is death. A total range of effective mechanisms to deal with the health of the aged or younger population groups, including general improvements in standards and styles of life, could, under the best of circumstances, increase the percentage of persons living a full life span and reduce the occurrence and impact of disease on the population. To expect a noticeable improvement in such measures in a relatively short time from one government-sponsored program would be unrealistic. Additionally, if program efforts resulted in greater attention being paid to the health condition of the aged, it might increase the percentage of existing disease reported and give the image that these efforts to deal with the health problem had worsened the situation.

Program activities to deal directly with the health problems of the aged might alter circumstances noticeably in terms of disease and age subgroup-specific bed disability days or the morbidity/mortality ratio for specific causes. A program to increase the availability of medical care services or reduce barriers to needed utilization of such services would be likely to result in higher levels of use. Relating this increased use to measures of improved health might be difficult. On the other hand, the increased use itself and the lowered barriers, however these were addressed by the program, should be more easily assessed. Measures of health care services, resources, use, cost, and so on are available through various of the data collection activities of the NCHS. The Social Security Administration (and since the reorganization the Health Care Financing Administration) has issued periodic data on use and reimbursements under the Medicare program.

Policy Formulation and Program Development

The development of policy in the area of health insurance for the aged traces its history to earlier attempts to deal with the health needs of the population. In considering policy formulation and program development for the Medicare program, we have reviewed these prior efforts. This situation, where policy emerges over an extended period of time before the first passage of a major program, suggests difficulty in formulating a policy or in obtaining agreement on the direction it should take. The result, for health policy in the United States, has been long and continuing debate over the focus of that policy. The 1965 amendments to the Social Security Act that authorized both Medicare and Medicaid provided a limited and temporary resolution of the policy debate by establishing programs aimed explicitly at financing the medical care use of carefully defined segments of the population. This approach was a compromise between those who wanted far less in the way of a formal government program in the area of health care and those who wanted wider population coverage and for whom an explicit purpose was to bring about changes in the health care delivery system.

Recreating the intent of policy makers over a time span or tracing the development of a specific program requires interpretation and extrapolation from the statements and actions of individuals and consideration of the writings of others concerned with the issue. The positions taken by various individuals and organizations as expressed in statements, hearings, reports, and commentaries are a valuable source of information about the policy formulation process and the compromises it entailed.

Review of the legislation itself, the implementing regulations, and additional amendments provides a history of the program and the changes that have occurred in it in the years since it was instituted. Explicit policy pronouncements are less common after initial program authorization legislation has been passed. Presumably routine program "adjustments," however, can have substantial although possibly not easily recognized implications for policy. Review of these various items is necessary for an assessment of whether the program as implemented initially and as changed over time is consistent with the original policy intent.

Model Analysis

Assessing the relationship among problem, policy, and program in the attempts to deal with the health needs of the aged through Medicare requires the analysis of data not collected for this specific purpose. The analytic framework used was applied after the fact to routine data collected to monitor the performance of the program, and to specific data from the study designed to provide a limited assessment of the impact of Medicare. The policy implications drawn from the data and analysis, as a result, are beyond what was originally intended in the use of this material.

The Medicare program was designed to defray the costs of medical care for those over 65. Nevertheless, implicit in the entire effort was a desire to use this mechanism to improve the distribution of needed services to the aged and to upgrade the quality of medical care available to this population group. At the inception of the program, it was difficult to estimate the effect Medicare might have on the availability of health services for the aged, utilization of these services among the aged, personal expenditures for medical care by the aged, or the system for delivery of health services. Certain aspects of the impact of Medicare can be assessed best from national data and indexes concerning, for example, the financial burden of medical care of the aged, the economics of health care, the utilization of health services by the aged, and the availability of specific services and facilities. Such national data as are available in these areas come from program sources and the surveys conducted by the NCHS. However, changes in the way health care needs are defined, services are delivered, and facilities are developed, used, or coordinated can most effectively be assessed by more detailed studies of various parts of the medical care system. The delivery of medical care is organized primarily locally, to serve a local population. While there may be national trends and standards, the delivery and receipt of care are also local problems.

To assess the impact of Medicare on the provision and use of health care services from this perspective, a before-and-after study was undertaken in five selected midwestern communities, starting in 1966. One of the major objectives of this study was to determine the response of the health care delivery system to the financial mechanism of Medicare as it functioned to deliver needed care to the residents of communities and metropolitan areas. In the data analysis Medicare was viewed as a possible source of change in the way health services were delivered. The central concern was whether this payment mechanism did in fact stimulate the medical care delivery system to change in the direction of providing services more appropriate to the health needs of the aged population. In each of the communities studied, the medical services and facilities available to serve the Medicare population were viewed as a potential system that might or might not function as a set of interrelating parts in the delivery of health services to the residents of the community. Of concern was whether the medical care system would respond to the greater availability of funding for health services for the aged by concentrating its efforts on developing or improving those services and facilities most responsive to the unique needs of the aged, or would use these resources on services and facilities of a more general nature. Since the aged use a disproportionate share of virtually all relevant medical care facilities, such action would not necessarily have constituted a warping of the latent intent of the Medicare program, that is, improving the distribution and upgrading the quality of medical care available to the aged. However, it would have provided an upgrading of what was probably the most neglected area of care for the aged—care of the chronically ill through comprehensive services of a long-term nature.

Among possible consequences of the Medicare program, it was hypothesized that:

1. Community health care organizations would adjust to the expected increase in demand for services by shifting present resources of space, equipment, and personnel.
2. Eventually, there would be a reorganization of health resources (including the supply of doctors) to provide for better coordination and distribution of services demanded by older patients with predominantly chronic diseases.
3. Physicians, as the key to success or failure in implementation of the program, would work to improve the service capabilities of their organizations.
4. Older people would begin to alter the norms regarding the definition of appropriateness of seeking professional care and would increase their utilization of physicians.

The five communities studied were chosen to represent different types of cities and different levels of health and medical care services. The metropolitan community of Kansas City, Missouri, and its surrounding counties in the metropolitan area had the fullest range of services. Two cities of intermediate size (about 100,000 population) were studied. One had a well-developed medical community but no relationship with a medical school; the other had a more traditional organization of medical services and was associated with a medical center. The two smaller communities acted as medical care trade centers for local counties, but with somewhat different emphases. One was comparatively well endowed with medical services, while the other was a more medically impoverished area.

Methodologically, the investigation pursued parallel lines of inquiry. One was a study of community providers of health care services and their organization. Hospitals, extended care facilities (ECFS), nursing homes, home health services, physicians, and other manpower sources in the community were studied. The other line of inquiry was a study of the attitudes and utilization patterns of older persons through a household interview survey of random samples of more than 2,000 people aged 60 and over in the five communities. The group aged 60–64 was considered the control group for subjects chosen in the study who were 65 or older and eligible for benefits from the Medicare program. Data for both lines of inquiry were gathered in 1966 at the time the Medicare program began, in 1968 after the program had been operating for two years, and again in 1971.

Independent but comparable samples of people aged 60 and over were drawn for the first two surveys. The follow-up survey of older people in 1971 was done only in Kansas City and not in the other four communities. Evaluation of the earlier surveys indicated there were few differences among communities in orientation to Medicare, utilization patterns, or attitudes toward practitioners or resources. Since earlier samples from Kansas City were sufficiently large for comparison purposes, conducting the follow-up household survey in 1971 only there seemed appropriate.

Data on the community services were drawn from interviews with directors and administrators of community facilities, from interviews with a sample of practicing physicians (for 1971, 55 physicians in Kansas City and 135 in total were studied), and from secondary sources such as census reports and publications from official agencies or organizations. Since the earlier data did show considerable variation among communities in the availability of health services and in the development of home health services and extended care facilities after the introduction of Medicare, the 1971 follow-up study continued the collection and analysis of data from providers in all five communities. One minor variation from the earlier survey initiated in 1971 was that some physicians were interviewed while others completed a comparable questionnaire. Pretest results indicated the only significant difference between the two methods of collecting information was a higher completion rate with interviews. However, this method also required a greater investment of time and funds. Minor changes in the other schedules were also made to eliminate some questions or to update referents. Questions relating to comprehensive health planning programs, initiated between 1968 and 1971, were added to all the later schedules. Minor changes were also made in the household interview schedule. A few questions were dropped and a few altered to bring them up to date.

The analysis of data focused on social change; change in attitudes, beliefs, and behavior of providers and utilizers; and change in the organization and provision of health services in each community. The goal was to determine the possible consequences that an innovation in the method of paying for medical services might have for the attitudes and reported behavior of providers and consumers. Thus, 1971 information on providers' attitudes toward Medicare, their beliefs about the consequences of Medicare, their planning and decision-making processes, and the outcomes of those decisions in organizational settings was compared with responses from 1966 and 1968. Common to all groups was a series of questions about the effect of coordinative efforts of comprehensive health planning agencies.

For data from the household sample of older people, a direct evaluation of change (for Kansas City only) can be made. That is, responses to questions about perception of health status, illness orientations and behaviors, utilization of resources, and attitudes toward Medicare, hospitals, and physicians were collected in 1966 before the program was fully under way, again in 1968, and once more in 1971. Since the questions were the same and the respondents similar in each survey, it is possible to see some trends toward change in these areas.

2

HEALTH STATUS
OF THE AGED AND THE
HEALTH CARE SYSTEM
BEFORE MEDICARE

This chapter describes the nature and extent of the *problem* of health care of the aged, first of the three elements in the analytic perspective outlined in Chapter 1. What the evidence will show is that before 1966 (when Medicare began), the elderly in the United States had the greatest health care needs and the fewest resources to meet these needs. Lack of resources included lack of personal resources as well as insufficient access to community resources. In detail, then, we wish to review (1) the health status and health needs of the elderly up to 1965; (2) the resources available to meet health needs; and (3) the levels of use of care resources by the elderly.

HEALTH STATUS OF THE ELDERLY

As an initial step, the scope of the problem must be estimated in terms of the number of elderly to be considered. Some data comparing the elderly with the total U.S. population are shown in Table 2.1. It is clear that there has been a rapid growth in the absolute numbers of aged, as well as in the proportion of the total population the aged make up. What is shown in Table 2.1 represents an acceleration of changes that began around 1900. Moreover, during the decade beginning in 1960, the group 65 and over became the fastest-growing segment of the population, with a 1.9 percent increase between 1960 and 1970. It may be seen also that the median age of the total population began to increase after 1970 and is projected to continue in that direction well beyond 1980 (Siegel, 1979).

Changes within the aged population are further delineated in Table 2.2. The trend has been toward some decline in the proportion of "young-old," aged 65-69, and a corresponding increase in the percentages of "old-old," age

TABLE 2.1: Selected Trends of Population Age 65 and over

	1950	1960	1965[a]	1970	1974	1980[b]
Total U.S. population (in millions)	152.3	180.7	192.8	204.9	211.9	225.7
Total population 65 and over (in millions)	12.4	16.7	18.4	20.1	21.8	24.5
Percent of total 65 and over	8.1	9.2	9.5	9.8	10.3	10.9
Median age in United States	30.2	29.4	28.6	27.9	28.6	30.3

[a]Estimated.
[b]Projected maximum.
Source: U.S. Bureau of the Census, *Current Population Reports*, 1975.

80 and over. As we shall see later, the declines in the birth rate and infant mortality rate have resulted in an expansion in the proportion of all elderly. Declines in death rates have contributed to an extension of the average length of life, through an expansion of the number of those who survive to very old age. This is the group most at risk for health problems and least able to meet those needs.

Measurement of Health Status

Estimating the health status and health needs of the elderly is difficult to do with precision. One approach is to use relatively objective indicators such as diagnoses, findings from laboratory evaluations, and other medical results

TABLE 2.2: Percentage Distribution of the Aged Population

Age (in years)	1950	1960	1965[a]	1970	1976	1980[b]
65–69	40.7	37.2	36.4	35.0	36.1	34.9
70–74	27.8	28.6	27.9	27.2	25.8	27.3
75–79	17.4	18.5	18.9	19.2	17.7	17.3
80–84	9.3	9.6	10.5	11.5	11.9	11.3
85 and over	4.8	5.6	6.3	7.1	8.6	9.2
Totals	100.0	100.0	100.0	100.0	100.0	100.0
Number (millions)	12.4	16.7	18.4	20.1	22.9	24.5

[a]Estimated.
[b]Projected maximum.
Source: U.S. Bureau of the Census, *Current Population Reports*, 1975.

that can be obtained through study of a sample of medical records. However, this gives information only on a *treated* population, that is, only those patients who were sick enough to come to the facility for help. These data tell us nothing about the health status of the elderly in the community who did not seek care. In addition, the accuracy and completeness of recorded data vary from one source to another and may not always be comparable.

Another way to assess the health status of a particular group is through personal interviews conducted with representative samples of persons in the community. Questions about experiences with symptoms of illness, disability conditions, and global perceptions of health result in a subjective evaluation of health status. These data may or may not correspond to a medical definition of illness, and they are subject to distortion from imperfect recall and unreliability (Larson, 1978). Nonetheless, an individual's perception of his or her health often tells us more than knowledge of pathology about how that person will act in response to illness.

A third approach to measuring health status makes use of data both from records and from personal interviews. Relatively complete and reliable demographic information on deaths can be obtained from death certificates, although determining causes of death is more subject to error. National surveys of large samples of persons have produced reliable information on symptoms, diagnoses, physiological health, and perceived health, as well as reported use of medicines, doctors, and hospitals.

National reporting of statistics from hospitals and other institutions also provides a better picture of utilization of services. These data provide information for comparing groups on outcome dimensions (such as mortality, morbidity, disability, impairment, and average life expectancy) relative to input factors (such as doctor visits, hospital days of care, use of medications, immunizations, and so on). These variables also differ with respect to reliability and validity, but are most commonly used to compare groups by age and other demographic and social variables. This was specifically the case for defining the health status of the elderly in describing the problem considered here before 1965.

Life Expectancy

Some illustrative data, shown in Table 2.3, indicate that average length of life at birth had continued to increase, an extension of a trend beginning in the early 1900s. It may be seen also that women, especially white women, maintained a sizable advantage in years of life over men in the same racial group. The average life expectancy at 65, that is, the number of years of life remaining to someone who is at 65 years of age, however, suggests a much narrower advantage in years of women over men and of white over nonwhites. Furthermore, unlike the average for life expectancy at birth, the

**TABLE 2.3: Average Life Expectancy
(in years)**

	At Birth			At Age 65		
	1900	*1950*	*1965*	*1900*	*1950*	*1965*
All persons	42.0	68.2	70.2	—	—	—
White males	48.0	66.5	67.6	12.0	12.8	13.0
White females	51.0	72.2	74.7	12.0	15.0	16.6
Nonwhite males	33.0	59.1	61.1	10.0	12.8	13.0
Nonwhite females	35.0	62.9	67.4	11.0	14.5	15.8

— = not available.

Source: Department of Commerce, *Statistical Abstract of the United States,* Washington, D.C., 1967.

number of years of life at age 65 had increased by only a few years since 1900, virtually no improvement at all (Coe, 1973). The implication is that increased average life expectancy is due primarily to successes in reducing infant mortality and childhood diseases and much less to effective control of diseases affecting the elderly. The infant mortality rates, that is, the deaths of infants under one year of age, had been dramatically reduced through better prenatal care, improved nutrition, rising standards of living, and successes in combating infectious diseases. Consequently, more infants survived to adulthood. However, similar successes had not been achieved in combating chronic conditions, which become more prevalent after age 35. Hence, life expectancy for older adults had improved very little.

The ratio between males and females in the 65-and-over age group in this country has shifted appreciably during this century. There were equal proportions of aged males and females through the 1930 census. This ratio dropped to 90 males per 100 females by 1950, and 83 males per 100 females by 1960. By 1975, there were 69 males for every 100 females 65 and over. For those 75 and over, there were 83 males per 100 females, in 1950, and 58 males per 100 females by 1975.

Not only did the aged make up a larger proportion of the population of the United States by the mid-1960s, growing from 3 percent in 1900 to 9.5 percent in 1965, their age group had also become predominantly female. It was quite apparent that the size and percentage of the population 65 and over had grown considerably in the several decades before the passage of Medicare, but that the group was largely female may have been less apparent.

Mortality

Rates of mortality, that is deaths, had been declining slowly since 1900. Total deaths per 1,000 population stood at 9.4 in 1965, a decline from 9.6 in

TABLE 2.4: Mortality per 1,000 Population

Age Group	1950	1965
65–74	49.3	50.5
75–84	104.3	98.2
85 and over	216.4	212.8

Source: Department of Commerce, *Statistical Abstract of the United States*, Washington, D.C., 1967.

1950. For the elderly, there was a parallel decline, with some variations, as indicated in Table 2.4. Of equal concern to planners in 1965 were the causes of death. For males and females over age 65, six of the ten leading causes of death were from chronic diseases: heart disease, cancer, stroke, diabetes, emphysema, and cirrhosis of the liver. The others of the ten leading causes were pneumonia (number 4), accidents (number 5), suicide (number 9), and homicide (number 10). Heart disease, cancer and stroke accounted for about 85 percent of all deaths.

Morbidity and Disability

Data from many studies have consistently shown that the elderly have more chronic diseases and more disability from diseases. The incidence of acute illnesses and of injury is lower among the elderly, but recovery from acute illness and injury is slower than for younger age groups. Some illustrative data for 1964 from the National Center for Health Statistics are shown in Table 2.5.

TABLE 2.5: Selected Dimensions of Disability and Injury

	Rates per 100 Persons		
	Total	Under 65	65 and over
Restricted activity days per person per year	16.3	17.0	38.4
Bed disability days per person per year	6.1	6.0	14.0
Activity limited by chronic conditions (percent)	12.5	12.4	48.8
Incidence of acute conditions per 100 persons	210.6	241.3	136.9*
Persons injured per 100 persons	38.7	27.5	17.0

*45+ years and over.

Source: Department of Commerce, *Statistical Abstract of the United States*, Washington, D.C., 1967.

EVALUATION OF RESOURCES

Health Resources

Evaluation of the adequacy of health resources required looking at two principal dimensions, availability and accessibility. Availability refers to the actual presence of different kinds of services, and this is a reflection of the purpose of the facility. Thus, even among health resources such as hospitals, there was specialization according to disease or type of case (such as tuberculosis, mental diseases, or maternity cases) or by population (such as pediatrics, adult care, or geriatrics). The community general hospital provided a wide range of services to most of a community's population, but even here the emphasis was on acute care services rather than rehabilitation and long-term care. That is, hospitals were organized and medical staffs were trained to respond to acute episodes of disease that can be treated quickly. The expectation was that the patient can recover fully in a very short time. These hospitals were not organized to deal effectively with chronic, disabling conditions that required some supervision and surveillance over a prolonged period, perhaps even for the lifetime of the patient.

Accessibility refers to the location or distribution of services in a community. There were obvious differences in accessibility for rural and urban populations, since most services were located in urban areas. Rural residents had to travel much further to obtain specialty services when they were needed. Even within urban centers, however, health services were relatively inaccessible to populations such as the inner-city poor and other disfranchised groups without access to adequate public transportation. The elderly were often in these groups, especially in large cities in which private health providers, that is doctors, hospitals, and ambulances, had relocated in suburban and exurban areas populated by younger families. This left the underfinanced municipal health systems to provide care for the poor and elderly who remained in the city (Shonick, 1979).

Some data presented in Table 2.6 illustrate the trends in growth of selected institutional services prior to 1965. It is instructive to compare short-term hospitals with long-term hospitals in light of the trend for all hospitals (including specialty institutions). The trend for all hospitals between 1950 and 1965 was toward a slight increase in number of institutions (5 percent), with a larger jump in number of beds (17 percent) and, therefore, in average size of institutions. This growth outstripped the "need" as measured by utilization, since occupancy rate (the average percentage of beds filled each day) declined despite a reduction in the number of beds per 1,000 population.

It is apparent that most of this growth was due to huge increases in short-term (acute) care facilities. For these facilities, the number of institutions and the number of beds increased at a rate nearly three times that for

TABLE 2.6: Selected Characteristics of Hospitals, 1950 and 1965

Characteristics	1950	1965	Percent Change
All hospitals			
Number of hospitals	6,788	7,123	4.9
Number of beds (0005)	1,456	1,704	17.0
Number of beds per 1000 population	9.6	8.9	–7.3
Occupancy (percent)	86.0	82.0	–4.6
Nonfederal short-term			
Number of hospitals	5,031	5,736	14.0
Number of beds (000's)	505	741	46.7
Number of beds per 1000 population	3.3	3.9	18.2
Occupancy (percent)	74	76	2.7
Nonfederal long-term			
Number of hospitals	412	283	–31.3
Number of beds (000's)	70	66	–5.7
Number of beds per 1000 population	—	—	—
Occupancy (percent)	86	85	–1.2

— = no data.

Source: Department of Commerce, *Statistical Abstract of the United States*, Washington, D.C., 1975.

all hospitals. Although the general population was not growing this quickly, occupancy rates still increased, if only slightly. This phenomenal growth was at the expense of long-term care resources, including mental hospitals and tuberculosis sanitoria. Here, the number of hospitals declined by nearly one-third and the number of beds per 1,000 population dropped slightly, indicating an increase in average size of institution. Occupancy rates, however, remained the same.

The nursing home industry began to grow after World War II, but had not yet shown the extraordinary rate of change that has characterized it in the 1970s. In 1964, before Medicare and Medicaid, there were about 15,000 nursing and personal care homes in existence. Altogether there were 576,000 beds in these homes and about 519,000 residents in them, an occupancy rate of 90 percent. Eight of ten homes were proprietary and more than three of five (64 percent) were small, that is, under 30 beds. Ninety-one percent of the patients were 65 or older. At the time of this report there were about 47 employees per 100 residents and an average monthly charge of $185.00 (NCHS, 1965c).

The relative costs of operating these facilities up to 1965 are shown in

TABLE 2.7: Selected Financial Data on Hospitals, 1950 and 1965

Characteristic	1950	1965	Percent Change
All hospitals			
Assets (millions)	$7,791	$24,502	214.5
Expenses (millions)	$3,651	$12,941	609.0
Personnel per 100 patients	84	139	65.5
Average cost per patient day	$7.89	$25.29	220.5
Nonfederal short-term			
Assets (millions)	$3,350	$12,476	272.4
Expenses (millions)	$1,523	$6,643	336.2
Personnel per 100 patients	191	252	31.9
Average cost per patient day	$15.62	$44.88	187.3
Nonfederal long-term			
Assets (millions)	$449	$998	122.3
Expenses (millions)	$117	$406	247.0
Personnel per 100 patients	57	115	101.8
Average cost per patient day	$5.39	$19.79	267.2

Source: Department of Commerce, *Statistical Abstract of the United States*, Washington, D.C., 1975.

Table 2.7. These data reveal consistent increases for all resources in assets, expenses, number of personnel (personnel was the single most expensive item), and cost per patient day. Of major concern, of course, were the increases in cost of services for the elderly, primarily long-term care.

Health manpower trends between 1950 and 1965 paralleled those for most health facilities, especially short-term hospitals. As indicated in Table 2.8, there were consistent increases in the ratio of physicians and nurses to population, but a slight decline in the proportion of dentists (which returned to 1950 levels by 1975). Not shown in the data are increases in ancillary personnel such as practical nurses (LPNs), midwives, and nursing aides.*

Other Resources

In addition to having greater health needs and less access to health

---

*Since 1965, the trends for all health resources have continued, except that the total number of hospitals and beds has declined. Costs have increased at double the rate of costs of other goods and services, while the 1960s "shortage" of both nurses and physicians has become an "average" predicted for the 1980s.

TABLE 2.8: Supplies of Certain Health Professionals, 1950 and 1965

Type	1950	1965
Physicians (per 1,000 population)	149	153
Dentists (per 100,000 population)	50	45
Nurses (per 1,000 population)	249	319

Source: Department of Commerce, *Statistical Abstract of the United States*, Washington, D.C., 1967.

resources, the elderly were at a disadvantage with respect to economic resources. In part this stems from the fact that for most people income is derived from employment, and most elderly are retired or otherwise unemployed. Then, too, retirement programs vary widely in adequacy of meeting the basic needs of older people. About 45 percent of the income of the elderly came from public sources, that is Social Security, veteran's benefits, and public assistance, with another third from earnings and 15 percent from investments. Contribution from relatives and miscellaneous made up the remaining 5 percent (Epstein and Murray, 1967)

Before 1965, the general economic situation for many elderly was particularly bleak. For example, in 1963, using a definition of poverty level, that is, a level below which minimum needs cannot be met, based on average housing rental amount and a food expenditure-total income ratio, the poverty level was estimated to be $1,800 for an elderly person living alone or $2,500 for an elderly couple. By these criteria, 65 percent of the 8.7 million unmarried persons age 65 or over had annual incomes below the poverty level and another 8 to 9 percent were described as "near poor." Married couples were only somewhat better off: 24 percent had incomes below $2,500 and another 17 percent were described as "near poor." Thus, although some elderly had assets such as a home or other property and some investments, the majority had little available cash to pay for needs beyond food and shelter.

Further, it should be noted that before 1965 the majority of the elderly lived independently in communities. This included about 75 percent of married couples and 60 percent of unmarried persons. Some comparisons between the living arrangements of men and women, as shown in Table 2.9, indicate that a majority of the men and about one third of the women were married and lived with their spouse in independent households. At the other extreme, only four percent of men and women were in institutions for the elderly (Epstein and Murray, 1967). Although the majority of households of the elderly had no adult children present, and the percentage increased with the age of the head of the household, most elderly in all age groups lived within an hour's travel time of their children, and 90 percent lived within one day's travel time of their children. Thus, family members provided social and emotional support although direct financial contributions were negligible.

TABLE 2.9: Living Arrangements of Elderly, 1963
(in percentages)

	Males	Females
Married, living with spouse	68	34
Unmarried, living with relatives	10	31
Unmarried, living alone or with nonrelatives	18	31
Institutionalized	4	4

Source: Epstein and Murray, 1967.

USE OF RESOURCES

Utilization of resources by the elderly changed little in the years before 1965 despite the increase in their numbers. A common indicator of patient-initiated utilization is the average number of contacts with physicians in one year. As can be seen from Table 2.10, there was a slight drop for all persons in the average number of physician visits per person from 1958–59 to 1963–64.

It is important to note the strong positive relationship between age and number of visits. This is often seen as indicating greater health care needs. Some additional data on physician visits by the elderly suggest that the relationship with age was stronger for whites than for nonwhites, and that older women generally had more physician visits than men, except for nonwhite women, whose contacts with doctors were much less frequent than for other groups (see Table 2.11). Other information about physician visits showed a strong positive relationship with level of income. Persons age 65 and over with incomes under $2,000 per year made 6.0 visits in 1963–64, compared with 8.5 visits per person with incomes of $10,000 or more. The contrasts are even sharper for those age 75 or more; 6.1 visits for those with incomes under $2,000 compared with 10.9 visits for those with incomes of $10,000 or more. Other interview data indicated that 30 percent of those over age 65 made no visits at all to physicians in 1962 and that 50 percent

TABLE 2.10: Physician Visits, per Person, by Age Group

	1958–59	1963–64
All ages	4.7	4.5
Under 14	4.7	4.2
15–24	4.0	4.3
25–44	4.7	4.5
45–64	5.1	5.0
65 and over	6.7	6.7

Source: National Center for Health Statistics, *Volume of Physician Visits, 1965.*

TABLE 2.11: Physician Visits, per Person, by Sex and Race, 1963–64

	White		Nonwhite	
	Male	Female	Male	Female
All ages	4.1	5.3	3.0	3.6
55–64	5.0	5.7	5.3	5.5
65–74	5.5	7.1	6.4	5.6
75 and over	7.1	7.8	6.3	3.5

Source: National Center for Health Statistics, Volume of Physician Visits, 1965.

reported not seeing a physician as often as they thought they needed to. By income level, 54 percent of men and 53 percent of women in the low-income third did not see a doctor as often as they should, compared with 42 percent of men and 36 percent of women in the highest-income third (Epstein and Murray, 1967).

Similarly, older people used more days of hospital care than did younger persons. In addition, the rates of admission and discharge were higher. For example, in 1964–65, the number of discharges from short-stay hospitals per 100 persons of all ages was 12.9. For those under age 17, the rate was 6.6; for those 45–64, 14.9; and for those 65 and over, 18.3. The average length of stay in days for the elderly was 13.1 days for each admission, compared with 4.5 days for children 1–14, and 9.9 days for adults age 45–64 (NCHS, 1965d).

Finally, we come to the issue of cost of obtaining care. Most of the elderly, like the majority of U.S. citizens, had some form of sickness insurance. Just before 1965, about 68 percent of all Americans were insured, as were 50 percent of those age 65 and over, with 64 percent of the aged who were married and 42 percent of those who were unmarried being insured. However, the elderly had less coverage than other groups did. For example, about 15 percent of those 65 or older had hospital insurance only, compared with 7 percent of all persons. Hospital and surgical plans were subscribed to by 71 percent of the elderly and 75 percent of all insured. Comprehensive plans that included payment for doctor visits covered 13 percent of the elderly and 17 percent of all persons. Health insurance also varied by perceived health status: 60 percent of the elderly who reported their health as good had some form of insurance compared to only 35 percent of those who reported their health status as poor (Epstein and Murray, 1967). The latter, however, used many more days of hospital care and physician services than the former.

Despite the insurance coverage they did have, older Americans paid a larger percentage of their annual incomes for health care and had more out-of-pocket expenses because of greater need and higher utilization of services than did the rest of the population. The magnitude of these expenses added to the growing economic burden on the aged. In 1962, for example, the average out-of-pocket cost of health care for all persons was about 5 percent of total family income. Out-of-pocket expenditures for health care were also under 5 percent for about one-third of married couples and unmarried females age 65 and over and for 50 percent of unmarried elderly males. However, 13 percent of couples and unmarried men and 20 percent of unmarried women had out-of-pocket expenses for medical care that equaled one-fourth or more of their annual incomes (Epstein and Murray, 1967).

Overall average health care expenditures were considerably higher for the aged than for other Americans. In 1962, the per capita cost for all health services was $119 for the total population and $244 for those age 65 and over (Feingold, 1966). Finally, it may be noted that the average cost for prescribed drugs in 1963 was $4 for those age 65 and over compared with $3.65 for those under age 65 (NCHSa).

DEFINING THE PROBLEM

In summary, while assessment of health status of various groups continues to occupy the attention of researchers, as yet no completely satisfactory procedure has been developed. Relatively objective measures such as diagnoses, test results, and other information from record audits are limited to treated populations and do not correlate well with reported behavior of patients. Subjective measures from interviews such as self-reports on symptom experiences and perception of health status are highly predictive of behavior in response to illness, but are subject to problems of reliability, validity, and recall (Larson, 1978). Frequently, comparisons among groups varying by age, sex, race, ethnicity, and social class are made on the basis of outcome variables such as life expectancy, rates of mortality and morbidity, and degrees of disability and impairment. Outcome measures such as these provide data that are more uniformly defined, collected under better controlled conditions, and, therefore, more comparable for different population groups. On the other hand, outcome measures are not strongly correlated with levels of utilization of medical care services. For example, despite the fact that the elderly use more medical services than people in younger age groups, life expectancy, that is, years of remaining life, has not increased appreciably since 1900 for people at age 65, although average life expectancy at birth has increased by nearly 50 percent in the same time period. Similarly, morbidity from chronic diseases and rates of disability and impairment continue to be higher for those 65 and over than for those in other age groups. The point is that it is difficult to assess the health status of the elderly and their resultant medical needs. Yet these data formed the basis for identifying the nature and scope of the problem at the time a national policy intended to provide for the health care needs of the aged was being considered.

It became apparent to advocates of change that the problem of health care services for the elderly had several dimensions. There was evidence that the number and proportion of elderly in the population were growing. It was also clear that the elderly had more health problems involving chronic diseases and disabling conditions. Thus, it was inferred that medical *need* was greater for the elderly than for other age groups and that the *demand* for services should be expected to be higher for this age group than for younger individuals. Another dimension of the problem, which seemed to counteract the prediction for higher demand by the elderly for health care, was the *cost* of services juxtaposed with the economic status of the elderly.

The rising costs of health services bore heavily on the elderly in the mid-1960s. Prior to 1965, almost half (45 percent) of persons aged 65 or over were classified as below the poverty level (compared with 14 percent in 1977). This disproportionately affected blacks and females living alone. Despite their impoverished status, most elderly persons lived independently in the community. Less than 5 percent of those over age 65 lived in nursing homes or other institutions. Only about 17 percent lived in families where they were not the head of the household. The rest lived alone or as head of a family. Even though most elderly maintained an independent existence, most had frequent contacts with adult children, siblings, and other relatives. In fact, then as now, family and neighborhood support networks played an important role in maintaining the independence of the elderly in the community (Shanas, 1979).

Despite social and family support, the concern for health and economic needs of the elderly continued to mount. While these trends showed clearly the increased availability of most health resources, for the elderly, whose major problems required more long-term, intermediate levels of care and less of the care provided in short-term facilities designed to deal with acute conditions, there was a *decrease in resources most appropriate to their needs*. At the same time, the costs of these services continued to escalate while economic resources of the elderly decreased. Rising costs, plus the trend for health care resources to be in urban and suburban areas, made services less accessible to the poor, in general, and the (poor) elderly most particularly.

At the time legislators were looking carefully at the increased needs of the elderly, the trends were toward fewer resources appropriate to the needs of the elderly, resources geographically located in areas that reduced accessibility to them and at a cost that was rapidly going to exceed the ability of older patients to pay for them even if they were available and accessible.

For many observers, the economic dimension was the most salient and, in many respects, the easiest one on which to obtain data. At the same time, there was considerable disagreement among members of Congress, the AMA, and other lobbying groups about interpretation of the data and, indeed, their validity. In general, the picture presented in legislative hearings was particularly bleak. For example, despite the greater medical need, the rates of utilization of services were higher, but not proportionately so. At the same time, the implication from other data was that financial limitations served as a restraint on the level of utilization of services by the aged.

The problem of the health status of the elderly and how to solve that problem obviously could be defined and approached from more than one perspective, which legislators had to consider. As noted above, possible concerns included the emphasis on acute care services, availability and accessibility of appropriate services when needed, and how to pay for the services. Despite its multifaceted nature, the problem of health care for the elderly, after much debate and bargaining, was finally defined for policy purposes as a *lack of ability by the elderly to purchase medical services.* The issue of concern was the potential financial barriers to receipt of health care services among the aged. This relatively narrow focus had several important implications for the policy formulated and the program developed.

An economically oriented approach to policy was seen as most appropriate. That is, it seemed that a suitable policy would provide a mechanism to relieve the aged of the burden of meeting the costs of care. Only implicitly was there consideration of broader aspects of delivery of services. The problem was viewed in terms of the adverse financial position of the aged, coupled with their lower levels of health insurance coverage, both in numbers covered and benefits provided, and their higher levels of need for and use of care as compared with younger members of society. This approach to the problem set the stage for an attempt to deal with it solely in terms of the ability of the elderly to pay for care, but did not open the way for consideration of more basic issues in the organization and distribution of medical care. However, a focus on medical care, rather than health care, delimited possible policy and program boundaries. Defining the problem form the perspective of the ability to pay for needed medical care services did not address any of these other aspects of the health or medical care needs of the elderly. At best, there could be an implicit assumption that normal market forces would deal with these other aspects of the care needs of the elderly as a result of the influence on supply of an improved purchasing power.

The definition of the problem of the health of the aged from an economic perspective facilitated placing it within an established framework of limited responsibility for its solution on the part of the government. Society at large accepts the concept of the need to provide a measure of income replacement for the lost earning capacity of those of retirement age, without

accepting blame for the social condition of the aged. These income maintenance benefits provide a floor of income for the aged and also help maintain
the stability of the economy as a whole. Health care could be viewed and
approached in the same way. The aged could be provided with health
insurance to cover some, but not all, of the costs of care. The use of needed
services could be encouraged without directly dealing with problems of care
delivery by providing benefits only as a payment or reimbursement for
actual utilization.

An attempt to restructure the delivery system for medical care or to
alter the basic mechanism for care financing would have had to address more
universal aspects of the problems of health care for the whole population,
rather than just those aspects related to the ability of the elderly to finance
their care needs. Such an approach would have had to deal more directly
with the societal responsibility for satisfying the right of all members to
health care.

It is important to note that Medicare was not the only result of the policy based on the definition of the problem in terms of ability to pay for care.
The Medicaid program was also authorized by the 1965 amendments to the
Social Security Act, but under Title XIX. As was mentioned earlier, Medicaid follows the social welfare tradition in that it employs a means test as
contrasted to the universal approach of the Medicare program. Those aged
65 and over who are recipients of Supplemental Security Income or are otherwise in financial need can receive Medicaid benefits. The program was
added to serve the poor regardless of age, but for many reasons, its impact
was not entirely positive (Stevens and Stevens, 1974). Through the two programs as established in 1965, the aged, and certain other specified categories
of persons, obtained some measure of relief from the burdens of the cost of
medical care. For Medicaid, because of the conception of the financial inca-
pacity to meet medical care costs, those eligible for the program received
covered services with no need to pay part of the bill. For Medicare, the program required partial payment by the beneficiary.

Before we move to a discussion of the development of Medicare, let us
review briefly the implications of some alternate definitions of the problem.
There are at least three different ways in which the health problem of the
aged could have been defined. According to one definition of the problem,
the aged not only suffered from a financial difficulty in meeting the costs of
medical care without some sort of special assistance, but also had unique
health problems related to chronic disease and aging that require special attention. This special attention could have been provided through coordinated, comprehensive care and health maintenance programs especially for
the aged, but this would have required substantial changes in the way medicine was practiced.

A second problem definition would have viewed the aged as one segment of society in general and considered the potential financial barrier to receipt of medical care for any citizen as the appropriate conception of the problem. This approach would have focused on the financing of medical care as the primary issue, as do Medicare and Medicaid, but would have taken the entire population as the base for concern, and not just the aged and indigent. Some of the proposals that have been put forward for national health insurance in the United States start from this definition of the problem, and attempt to establish a policy and program of publicly assured insurance for medical care costs.

The problem could have been defined from a third, even broader, perspective. It could have been viewed as the need of all citizens for access to health care; thus, policy would have been on the overall issue of control over the organization and delivery of health care services, including, but not limited to, the financing of such care. A definition of this nature, in 1965, would have been a major jump from the prevailing social values in health and health care in this country, which were not oriented toward control over the delivery system or over the individual practitioner beyond licensure.

Examples of these two more comprehensive approaches toward the problem of health care for the population are commonly found in other parts of the world. In most industrial nations, the problem of health care of the aged is dealt with in policy directed to the general issue of satisfying national health care needs for the entire population. Rather than providing a separate program of delivery or financing of health care for the aged, a national health system includes this aspect of medical care as one part of the whole.

For example, by 1965 Great Britain had already had nearly 20 years of experience with a more comprehensive, systemic approach to solving the problem, but the potential lessons to be learned from the British experience were ignored in the United States. The National Health Service (NHS) in Great Britain, established in 1948, is an example of an alternate approach to dealing with the problem of health care organization, delivery, and financing, not just for the aged or the indigent but for the entire population. This approach rests on a broader problem definition. The express primary purpose of the NHS was to eliminate the financial barrier to obtaining medical care and permit all persons in need of such care to obtain it without regard to cost. Two additional goals were to provide comprehensive care to meet all the health needs of each person and to adjust the distribution of services to the distribution of persons in need of those services (Coe, 1978).

To achieve these goals it was necessary to institute a major reorganization of the administrative offices of the Ministry of Health and of the operation of the hospitals and clinics. Physicians are paid by the NHS and hospitals are nationalized. This "balanced hospital community" involves coordination of ambulatory care in the community with a full range of institutional services including acute care, rehabilitation, and prolonged (that is, custodial) care (McKeown, 1964). This new system was not substituted for the fee-for-service system without disagreement. However, on most dimensions of health "outcome" measured at about the time Medicare was first instituted, which was approximately 20 years after the NHS was started, the data for Great Britain (England and Wales only) indicate more favorable circumstances there than in the United States. In 1966, there were 23.3 infant deaths per 1,000 live births in the United States; in Great Britain there were 19.2. Life expectancy at birth was 70.2 in the United States in 1965; in Great Britain it was 71.1. In 1968, the United States spent 7.5 percent of its national income on health care; Great Britain spent 5.2 percent. In the late 1960s, there were more physicians, nurses, and dentists per 1,000 population in the United States than in Great Britain, but more hospital beds per 1,000 population in Great Britain than in the United States. However, at the same time, there was more use of hospital care in terms of both admissions and days of care per 1,000 population in the United States, and more use of ambulatory care in terms of number of physician visits per year per person in Great Britain (Coe, 1978; Anderson, 1972). It is highly probable that the differences between Great Britain and the United States in social and cultural characteristics account for some of the differences in health care patterns noted. But it is interesting to note that in Great Britain ambulatory care (rather than in-patient care) is more common than it is in the United States, and that in addition a smaller percentage of resources is spent on health care in Great Britain. Hospital in-patient care is generally acknowledged to be the most expensive form of medical care. This is a useful point to bear in mind when considering the data to be presented later on the changes in cost, patterns, and levels of use of health care services that accompanied Medicare.

In the final assessment, it is obvious that the problem could have been defined much more grandly than it was. In fact, it could have been seen as a failure of the health care delivery *system*. Many "intermediate" definitions also were possible; these include lack of facilities to care for chronic diseases and a need for better geographic distribution of primary care services. In terms of our analytic perspective, the problem was poorly defined and this will influence the "goodness of fit" between problem and policy as formulated.

3
POLICY AND
PROGRAM DEVELOPMENT

The articulation of a policy and subsequent development of a program to solve a recognized social problem depends greatly on an accurate definition of the cause or causes of the problem. A mistaken definition of the problem can result in policy intentions that are also wide of the mark. Any program for remedial action, even one that accurately reflects the policy, is unlikely to resolve the problem adequately under these conditions. This is our general thesis with respect to the Medicare program. As we have just seen in the previous chapter, the problem of providing health care for the elderly was complex. The elderly, especially the poor elderly, were found to have the greatest health and medical needs, but to have had the fewest resources to meet those needs. The health care system in the United States was oriented primarily to doctor-dominated and hospital-based acute care services for episodic illnesses, and tended not to be appropriate for the chronic, disabling, but not life-threatening, problems of older people.

The complexity of the problem would seem to preclude a simple definition, yet the demands for action required a political compromise that could be translated into a policy-oriented program. In the case of Medicare, the issue was resolved by defining the problem primarily in economic terms; that is, what was identified as the most important factor was that older people seemed to be less able to pay for health and medical care. Therefore, a program to help them pay would be in order. However, the policy that would provide the framework for program specifics was complicated by several important assumptions or beliefs. One of these assumptions, now being seriously challenged (Knowles, 1977), was that more medical care would lead to improved health. That is, there was an uncritical acceptance of the effectiveness of modern medical care; thus, it was thought that a program to enable people to obtain more care would be beneficial. For acute, life-threatening diseases, such an assumption may have some merit. For chronic,

41

long-term conditions, that assumption has much less value. Second, health care of the elderly was narrowly defined in terms of medical and nursing care, excluding broader mental health and social, psychological, and environmental factors. Again, this results from the emphasis of modern medicine on acute disease and the lack of emphasis on chronic, disabling conditions, in which social and psychological factors are even more salient than they are in acute problems.

A third complicating factor involved disagreement on the philosophical underpinnings of the program that would affect the extent of support and how support would be provided. The principal factor in the disagreement was whether financial support was an earned right or welfare. Some felt that the aged had earned financial support by contributing to the economy through a lifetime of work. The contributions of workers were considered sufficient to provide for the small minority who had not been gainfully employed during their lifetime. This is similar to the insurance practice of using pooled resources (or premiums) to protect a larger group. Opponents, however, felt that working a lifetime did not automatically entitle anyone to services that were subject to economic rules of the market place. Rather, people should be concerned enough about retirement and health in their old age to have prepared for it during their working life through voluntary savings and insurance. These and other elements in our belief system that influenced the development of a policy and finally the Medicare program are described in this chapter.

FORMULATION OF A POLICY

The disagreement on philosophy just described provided the focus for much of the controversy in Medicare because it became articulated in terms of the *right* to health and, therefore, to adequate health care. At the present time, there is little question that most provider organizations subscribe to the belief that good health is a basic right. Even the American Medical Association, the most powerful of the private provider organizations and one that in the beginning resisted the Medicare program vigorously, adopted a bylaw stating that "it is the right of every citizen to have available to him adequate health care" (Harris, 1966). But before enactment of Medicare, consensus on this issue was much less clear.

Legitimation of the Right to Health

The above quotation, taken from the report on resolutions adopted by the House of Delegates of the American Medical Association in 1968, is a rather benign expression of a human right that is widely accepted today. Yet that simple statement masks a history of ideological confrontations that still exist with respect to means to an end, even if there is some agreement on the end itself. That is, there is general acceptance by health care providers and by the government of the right to good health and, therefore, good health care for all people regardless of their social or economic situation. However, there is not yet full agreement on how this right is to be protected and fulfilled. The development of the Medicare program is one expression of this continuing conflict.

In some respects, the concept of right to health has always been a part of the American philosophy, since the term appears in the equivalent of the *Congressional Record* in 1796 (Chapman and Talmadge, 1972). The expression of policy then, however, was both limited and quite explicit. It referred to the right of people to be protected from "certain health hazards" regardless of socioeconomic status. The health hazards of most concern included the epidemics of yellow fever, smallpox, and influenza that periodically ravaged communities in the newly formed nation. The focus, then, was on the people as a collective, not as individuals, a focus that found further expression in the development of the Marine hospital, a precursor of the present Public Health Service. It is important to remember, however, that *everyone* had that right, and that it was the government's responsibility to promote and protect that right.

For more than 100 years, until the 1920s in fact, neither this policy nor its expression was seriously challenged. During this period of national growth, the Public Health Service had grown, and the kinds of health needs and resources had also changed. Interestingly enough, during this period, the strongest support for increased government activity via the United States Public Health Service to protect the right to collective health came from the American Medical Association (AMA). The AMA often led the way toward formulation of programs to meet health needs of the population, such as the passage of the Food and Drug Act of 1905. In the 1920s, however, the AMA itself underwent a change in leadership, basically from control by academically oriented members to control by medical practitioners. One consequence was a reversal of many organizational policies and repudiation of some former positions on the government's role in the delivery of health care. This included a diminution in emphasis on the belief that health is a basic right, if not abandonment of the belief altogether (Chapman and Talmadge, 1972).

The reversal may in part be charged to some efforts in Congress and in the Public Health Service itself to extend the definition of the right to health to *individuals* as well as to individuals collectively although this application had never been a part of the general philosophy. It is easy enough to see that such a shift would have important economic consequences, not entirely deleterious, for medical practitioners. The medical profession is often charged with responding negatively as an organization principally on these economic grounds. As a matter of fact, the shift to a focus that was individual as well as collective also was contrary to the basic elements of a national philosophy of individualism. To the extent that ordinary citizens could articulate their beliefs, there probably would not have been widespread support for the notion that the government had a responsibility to protect a person's right to individual health care.

Before the economic depression of the 1930s, the prevailing political philosophy in the United States linked the moral stance of individual freedom with an economic preference for an unregulated market. That is, according to this philosophy, individuals had the right to be free to provide for themselves and their families according to their own capabilities, and the best chance for fulfilling their capabilities was provided by a free market economy. Those who failed to achieve success could turn to their families or to private charity for support. The government, however, had little role in the process except where it was recognized that conditions beyond the individual's control were hampering his or her pursuit of individual achievement. There was consensus that the government, with emphasis on local and state rather than federal government, had the obligation to intervene only when conditions were beyond control of the individual (Stevens and Stevens, 1974). Obviously, this philosophy does not differ markedly from earlier expressions limiting the right to health protection to epidemics of disease and environmental hazards.

The depression of the 1930s, however, placed a great strain on belief in the viability of the philosophy of individual achievement. That is, during the height of the depression, there were many able-bodied persons who were unemployed but willing and anxious to work. During this critical period there occurred a shift in philosophy from emphasis on individual rights to an emphasis on a stronger governmental role. The scope of the problem required intervention on a national level and only the federal government had the capacity to act effectively. The shift toward a stronger governmental role was not complete, of course. Indeed, the proper degree of government participation is still debated today. The compromise, however, included passage of the Social Security Act of 1935, which provided guarantees of a sort of income in old age in return for contributions made by the individual during his or her working life time. This "social insurance" approach was more palatable to individual rights advocates because it meant that the individual had "earned" this protection through participation in the labor force and was not being given "charity." Thus, the bill was finally passed and signed into law (Howards, Brehm, and Nagi, 1980).

The legitimacy of the right to health of the collective thus has never been in contention. The right to health of individuals has gained more legitimacy since the passage of the Social Security Act in 1935. It is our point, of course, that the amendments to that act in 1965 that included Medicare were a specific expression of the right to health even if limited to a particular age group. That limitation itself was a political and economic compromise. The passage and implementation of Medicare were an expression of the government's acceptance of its responsibility for insuring the right to health of elderly individuals. Insofar as the Congress represents the people, passage of the amendments indicated the people's acceptance of this legitimacy as well.

Acceptance by the people can be shown in ther ways as well. The idea of Medicare as insurance for older people was overwhelmingly approved by two-thirds of a regional sample in 1966 and almost nine out of ten in a 1971 sample from the same region (Coe and Peterson, 1973). More germane here, however, is the issue of national health insurance (NHI) that transcends age groups, economic status, or any other characteristic. Table 3.1 shows the public preference regarding various NHI plans, as shown in a recent survey of a nationally representative sample (Committee for National Health Insurance, 1975). Those favoring the third and fourth options were mostly younger, less affluent, and politically "liberal." Older people were more likely to choose the first option because they "already have an NHI plan." It is important to note that more than one in five respondents favored a program fully owned and operated by the federal government.

In another survey, this time conducted by Business Round Table, 59 percent of the more than 1,000 respondents indicated that some form of NHI was a good idea, despite the fact that 88 percent were already covered by some form of insurance. These respondents were further asked to indicate which type of plan they preferred according to control, payment mechanisms, and benefit levels. Most preferred a plan that was government-regulated, but operated by private insurance companies (48 percent). A substantial minority (29 percent) chose a plan that was regulated and operated by the government. Most respondents (50 percent) preferred a plan in which costs were shared by employer and employee or the government for the unemployed. About one-fourth preferred cost-payable deductions and

TABLE 3.1: Public Preference for Health Insurance Program

Program	Percent in Favor
Maintenance of current provisions	13
Catastrophic insurance for all and general medical insurance for poor	23
An NHI program that guarantees as much care as needed by anyone	35
A totally nationalized system in which care is guaranteed and the federal government takes over all resources and personnel	22
Other	7

Source: Committee for National Health Insurance, 1975.

general tax money supplements. The rest had no preference. Finally, 52 percent opted for full benefits without limits, while one-fourth chose plans with benefit limits, but options to pay for services beyond a benefit limit (Committee for National Health Insurance, 1975).

The perspective of providers varies on the legitimacy of the right to health and the government's responsibility to assure that right. The institutional providers seem to focus on the mechanisms of government participation rather than the appropriateness of its participation. Individual providers have taken various stances at different times, but there now appears to be a consensus that individuals have a right to health and good health care. The AMA represents the most powerful group of individual providers and takes the most conservative stand on that belief. Yet the House of Delegates did adopt the resolution that contained the statement quoted at the beginning of this chapter. That is at least prima-facie evidence that the right to good health is widely accepted and acknowledged.

Other Policy Assumptions

While a majority view now clearly supports the idea of the right to health, there has been less unanimity about how that right should be fulfilled. The principal arguments employed by major factions are discussed later in this chapter. Here we wish to note three other assumptions, related to the right to health, that were made by framers of the policy leading to the Medicare program. One assumption is that rights ought to be universally applied at least within this specified age group. Therefore, all the elderly should be eligible regardless of actual need or available resources. They argued that this was an earned right, not welfare, and that a means test to determine financial eligibility was inappropriate. In other words, if adequate health care was an earned right, then whether one was rich or poor, relatively healthy or sick was irrelevant, and a means test of the type typically used in welfare programs to determine eligibility was also irrelevant.

This is related to a second assumption, that for health care a service benefit program would be more appropriate than a cash benefit program. In other words, benefits would be payment or reimbursement for specific health services used rather than an amount added to a cash benefit that could be spent then for nonhealth as well as health items at the individual's discretion. This bases use of services on the need for medical care without concern for ability to pay, an approach which could affect even the well-to-do elderly.

"Cashing out" the anticipated additional financial assistance needed to cover the cost of medical care services would not have assured use of these services when needed. Providing the cash equivalent of the cost of various necessities such as food, clothing, and shelter is a common practice in public income maintenance programs. This is the system used in making benefits available independent of whether the amount provided is considered adequate to the need. The individual is then free to reallocate the benefits received as he or she sees fit or as necessity dictates. To avoid the possibility that any increase in cash benefits to cover the expected cost of medical care would be diverted to other purposes, this approach was not used in either the Medicare or the Medicaid program. Benefits were made available only for use for the item of interest. In Medicaid, a vendor payment plan was used where the individual is not involved in the financial transaction. The provider is reimbursed directly for services provided to an eligible recipient. In Medicare, the system is a modified vendor payment plan. Under Part B (Supplementary Medical Insurance), the individual will pay for medical services and be reimbursed by the program if the total bills in a year meet the standards for reimbursement, unless assignment, which will be discussed shortly, is used. The intent of this approach is to assure use of the medical services needed. In brief, Medicare does not fund needed medical care by increasing the monthly benefit level by an amount to cover average use but by providing partial payment for care actually received on a modified vendor payment basis.

Part of the rationale underlying this assumption was a belief by supporters that the elderly would seek care only for actual needs and not "abuse" the system by seeking professional services for "trivial" symptoms or for problems not related to health. This belief has received some empirical support that laid to rest the "economic man" hypothesis that was promoted before Medicare began (Coe and Associates, 1970; Munan, Vobecky, and Kelly, 1974). The "economic man" hypothesis holds that anything that is of value, free of cost, and readily available will be used whether needed or not. One argument against compulsory health insurance and subsidization of costs of health services was that older people would quickly increase use of valuable and "scarce" health services unnecessarily and inappropriately. Application of this hypothesis to Medicare ignored the fact that it was not "free"; that is, that there were premiums, co-insurance, and deductible provisions, as well as use of Social Security funds. It also ignored the wealth of research information indicating that utilization of health services is influenced by social and psychological factors, as well as economic ones, that would preclude an immediate rise in seeking of help by older people.

Finally, although not exhaustively, it was assumed that even a limited change would produce benefits, despite the recognition that the delivery of health services was part of a very complex system. As we have seen, the problem was defined *principally* in economic terms, although other factors were known. The solution was to provide financial support for the elderly, knowing that other parts of the system would be affected and would, in turn, exert influence in the financial realm. It was assumed, however, that these influences could be studied and controlled. Thus, the explicit intent of the legislation was to lower the financial barrier to health care for the elderly by a mechanism of health insurance. The implicit intent was to use payment provisions to encourage private and public providers to cooperate in developing a more comprehensive and integrated health care delivery system.

DEVELOPMENT OF THE PROGRAM

Legislative Background of Medicare

Beginnings

The passage of the Medicare program as part of the 1965 amendments to the Social Security Act of 1935, as a newly added Title XVIII, signaled a new era in compulsory social insurance for the United States. Although we were the last major industrialized nation to establish an insurance program of this type, the ideas of social insurance and compulsory benefits are not new even in the United States. The heritage of Medicare can be traced back more than 50 years before the 1965 passage of the program to the Progressive Party of Theodore Roosevelt, which, in 1912, first advocated government-sponsored health insurance. In fact, even before that, the American Socialist Party advocated a government-sponsored social insurance program like those developed in late nineteenth-century Europe. However, at that time, the idea had not received widespread attention (Myers, 1970).

Interest in social insurance, especially focused on health care for the whole population, did gain impetus through some legislative efforts and national investigations. One of the earliest of these was the bill sponsored by the American Association for Labor Legislation in 1912. This bill would have provided insurance against certain health risks for workers. Benefits were earnings-related and were to be paid for by contributions from the employee, the employer, and the state government. There was no federal participation proposed in this plan. It is of historical interest that this bill had the support of the American Medical Association in the early years. One AMA report at the time stated:

> Blind opposition, indignant repudiation, bitter denunciation of these laws is worse than useless . . . it leads nowhere and it leaves the profession in a position of helplessness if the rising tide of social development sweeps over it . . . in the end the social forces that demand these laws and demand an improvement in the social existence of the great mass of the people of the nation will indignantly force a recalcitrant profession to accept . . . (Harris, July 2, 1966, p. 30).

A half-century later these became prophetic words. By 1920, however, the AMA had changed its policy and its organizational philosophy and opposed social insurance in general and its compulsory provisions in particular. Perhaps more telling for this bill was the opposition of the leadership of the American Federation of Labor, on the grounds that emphasis on health insurance diverted attention from the major task of labor, to win higher wages. It might be added that this bill, along with much other domestic legislation, was lost because of the attention directed to events around World War I. The issue declined in importance during the prosperity of the 1920s.

A second important impetus toward social insurance for health care was the report of the Committee on the Cost of Medical Care. This was a bipartisan committee of professionals and interested lay persons, funded by several private foundations, which conducted an extensive study of the organization and costs of health services between 1927 and 1932. According to the committee's report, there was strong agreement that public health services and professional education should be strengthened. The members were divided on the role of (state) government in any health endeavor, but the majority did agree that group practice and voluntary insurance for medical care costs should be promoted (MacColl, 1966). The specter of the depression and subsequent social problems did much to reawaken interest in subsidized assistance for health care.

A third impetus, perhaps the most important, was the enactment of the Social Security Act of 1935, the 1965 amendments to which established Medicare and Medicaid. The development of the Social Security Act was briefly described in Chapter 1. What is important for Medicare is that the Social Security Act established (1) the principle of publicly funded contributory programs as an earned right under the social insurance provisions of the act; (2) a focus on the aged as one of the population groups of concern; and (3) federal financing of state-administered assistance programs. As we noted earlier, the strength of the value of individualism was significantly moderated by the depression of the 1930s. Many able-bodied and willing people could not support themselves because of events that were beyond their control. Hence, the need for a public program for the "deserving" disadvantaged was recognized and a program to provide financial support after retirement, based on an insurance concept of contribution during a work career, was promulgated.

From an economic perspective, it was apparent that certain groups were disadvantaged. Primarily, these were the elderly whose savings had been wiped out in the Great Depression and the very young, that is, dependent children, who could not be expected to contribute to their own support. Other groups included the disabled and blind. Priority for providing support, therefore, focused on these groups. Finally, the sheer size of the population needing help required participation of the federal government with its greater resources, either directly or through the states.

At the same time, but quite independently, a program of hospital insurance, begun in Texas in 1929, was rapidly developing in other states and finally would emerge as the Blue Cross program. Similarly, in disparate locations, groups of doctors began to band together to form medical groups. In early 1939, a measure called the National Health Bill was introduced into legislation in the Congress of the United States by Senator Robert F. Wagner, Sr., of New York. The bill called for matching federal and state funds for public health programs approved by the Social Security Board for services and supplies needed to prevent, diagnose, and treat illness and disability (Harris, 1966).

The AMA, along with several other groups, responded to these proposed innovations with a vigorous protest, at least initially. For the most part, the position of organized medicine against the proposals was based on a series of principles that over the years had been worked out by the doctors' organization. In particular, heavy reliance was put on those principles regarding the doctor-patient relationship, its successful operation only through free choice under market conditions, the imputed value of services paid for by one's own funds, and the right of professional people to charge what they feel their services are worth since, by definition, lay persons are unqualified to make such judgments. Eventually, the AMA came to accept the principle of *voluntary* health insurance and even created a program of its own (Blue Shield). However, the furor that arose from the negative stand by the AMA on the grounds of their principles, and that obviously were not shared by everyone, had the unfortunate effect of detracting from the real achievements of organized medicine in raising the standards of medical training and practice in this country. It also had the effect of further delaying the passage of any legislation, including the National Health Bill, and in this the AMA was aided by the fact that the situation was not yet right for such an innovation.

In the first place, the nation's attention and energies were devoted to the problems of the emergence of the war in Europe in 1939 and 1940 and, finally, our involvement in it. Secondly, many of the important social and demographic changes noted earlier had not yet made their full impact felt. Third, during the period before and during the war, the federal government was not a strong force for initiating health legislation, after "the 100 Days" of 1933 and the Social Security Act of 1935. Nonetheless, even during the early 1940s several lawmakers were interested in reviving Senator Wagner's original National Health Bill. Soon there emerged what came to be known as the Wagner-Murray-Dingell bill, which proposed compulsory insurance coverage for employees and Social Security beneficiaries, and voluntary participation by others. To offset criticisms of "socialized medicine," the proposal specifically provided for free choice of physician and permitted physicians the option of participating or not in the program. By late 1944, however, considerations of another presidential election overshadowed the issue, and the proposal never left the committee room.

During the period between 1935 and 1950, there were considerable state and national efforts to establish health insurance programs. Congressional activities in this area also increased during this period. Of special note, besides the Wagner-Murray-Dingell bill, was the Taft proposal to provide limited public assistance for medical care for the elderly. This was a forerunner of the Kerr-Mills bill, the basis of the present Medicaid program. The familiar opposition from organized medicine and the insurance industry effectively lobbied against any legislative action. However, all of this was overshadowed by the events of World War II. One significant shift in support for health insurance came from labor organizations, which focused on health care and other fringe benefits through collective bargaining during the war when wages were frozen. Consequently, by 1950 several comprehensive health programs were in existence and the demand for more programs and for increased insurance benefits rose rapidly (Myers, 1970).

Movement toward Enactment

The period from 1950 to 1965 involved almost continuous controversy over health insurance. It was an important period for health insurance legislation, in part because more or less continuous congressional hearings on programs of subsidized health care kept the issue alive and in the public view. More importantly, however, from the perspective of the processes of innovation, there were several significant events that to some degree paved the way for passage of the final bill. Detailed reports of this period are available elsewhere (Myers, 1970), and only a few key factors will be noted here. One of these was the 1951 report of President Truman's Committee on the Health Needs of the Nation. This report established that health was a basic right and that, under conditions then existing, many were being deprived of that right. The committee also recommended that federal support be provided through the mechanism established by the Social Security Administration. There were, of course, those who opposed this recommendation, but as an underpinning for the acceptability of later programs it proved to be a necessary if not sufficient first step.

A second factor, already noted above, was the increasing demand by labor unions for health care and insurance as part of the fringe benefits of employment. This greatly expanded the benefits available and the number of persons covered. Many of these unions and their leaders—the United Mine Workers and John L. Lewis, the United Auto Workers and Walter Reuther, and the Kaiser Foundation, among others—had become sponsors of highly sophisticated and successful mechanisms for providing health care services.

Third, the elderly became the focus of attention—in part because of greater needs and lesser resources, but also because payments through Social Security were seen as "earned" benefits and not "welfare."

The arguments for and against insurance for medical care, and over what population should be insured and under whose auspices, continued unabated throughout the period. By the beginning of 1960, the foundation was fairly well established for what was to be the final push for passage of a bill for compulsory health insurance. A Senate Subcommittee on the Problems of the Aged and Aging had been established. Several measures had been proposed. By 1960, however, the battle lines were fairly well drawn. Proponents were "liberal" members of Congress, labor unions, and senior citizens' groups. Opponents were "conservative" members of Congress, AMA leadership, the insurance industry, and professional groups like the American Hospital Association and the Blue Cross Association.

Studies in economics and the other social sciences added to the data available, and presented comparable kinds of conclusions about the real plight of the aged. Even the detractors—especially the AMA—helped the cause by using outmoded and irrelevant arguments without any constructive alternatives and, because of their continuous campaign, by keeping the issue in the public view. Perhaps most of all, the presidential campaigns of 1960 and 1964 served not only to demonstrate the need for a health insurance program and to marshal evidence to support the contention that only the federal government had the resources to carry out such a program, but to legitimate the government's claim for responsibility for it on the grounds of providing for the rights of all the citizens.

The substance of the arguments of proponents and opponents is outlined in Table 3.2. Clearly, there was little agreement on any dimension. Even basic data on the elderly could be interpreted to give different views of their health status and financial situation. Basic differences in philosophy about the role of central government and in understanding of human motivation are also apparent. Proponents generally emphasized dimensions of need for insurance protection in a program of sufficient scope to accommodate ever increasing numbers of elderly. Opponents emphasized the potential for runaway costs of such a program, stating that these costs eventually would demand more federal participation.

These basic philosophical elements of individual versus collective needs, and earned benefits versus "welfare" continued to order the debate in Congress during the last few years prior to passage of the bill. They were reflected in the 1957 Forand bill for hospital and surgical services along with nursing home care and in an administration bill in 1959 to encourage private carriers to participate with reinsurance from the federal government. Various other proposals made through 1960 also received no final action in Congress.

Two further proposals are of significance in the development of Medicare, although there were many subsequent modifications in Congress.

TABLE 3.2: Arguments Concerning Social Insurance Proposals

Dimension	Arguments by Proponents	Arguments by Opponents
Need for protection	Elderly most in need, least able to pay hospital costs or to buy insurance; most affected by inflation.	Many elderly are financially well-off; just increase cash benefits to the poor; cost of insurance will rise, too.
Scope of the problem, requiring a national solution (such as Social Security)	There are no adequate private programs available; federally sponsored and coordinated program is necessary; because of experience with OASDI, Social Security Administration is ideal.	More than half the elderly already have some form of insurance; need is not so great; OASDI experience with cash benefits not relevant to a proposed service benefit program
Financing by those in the labor force	Younger workers purchase insurance against their old age needs; obtain financial relief for care of their parents.	Younger workers with low incomes pay for older workers with higher incomes; some older people won't need assistance.

TABLE 3.2 (continued)

Dimension	Arguments by Proponents	Arguments by Opponents
Effect on doctors, hospitals, and third-party payors	Private insurance will be stimulated because patients prefer "own" providers; program will never become wholly nationalized.	Private companies can not compete with subsidized programs; hospital benefits will lead to unlimited expansion and to socialized medicine.
Effect on individuals	Reducing financial barriers may reveal greater need but cost estimates are accurate.	Free care will lead to excessive use of hospitals and increase costs further.

Source: Myers. R. J. *Medicare.* Irwin, 1970.

One proposal to amend the Social Security Act of 1935 was passed in 1960 and became known as the Kerr-Mills Law, named after its sponsors. The other was a proposal from the Kennedy Administration.

The Kerr-Mills bill greatly increased federal matching monies to the states in the form of vendor payments to providers for specific services rendered rather than cash payments to beneficiaries. The vendor payment concept is important because it represents a compromise in philosophical perspective and allowed a payment mechanism to be established. As discussed earlier, cash payments similar to those provided in public assistance programs can be and are spent for goods and services at the recipient's discretion. Since payments are generally inadequate to fill all basic needs, recipients must often choose among items to be purchased. Priority is seldom given to health care. While social insurance programs are universal and apply to everyone who meets eligibility criteria regardless of income or other resources, the concern was that the elderly might require help with meeting the costs of health services. Since the problem was defined as inability to pay for medical care, it was logical to decide on payments directly to providers for service as a way of insuring, first, that costs of needed medical care would not be a deterrent to obtaining such care; and, second, that funds would go *only* for medical care and not for needs not related to health.

It is important to note that Kerr-Mills did establish a new public assistance program of medical care for the elderly through state-administered programs. With some changes, Kerr-Mills, which provided payment for physician and dentist services, hospital care, nursing home care, and some ancillary services, became the Medicaid portion of the 1965 Amendments to the Social Security Act of 1935.

The other proposal, which came from the Kennedy Administration, provided in its 1961 version for hospital and nursing home care, home health services, and out-patient care. There were some exclusions and there was a provision for co-insurance and deductibles. This bill underwent considerable change by amendments in 1962, 1963, and 1964 to expand benefits. Even after the 1964 national election, with its huge margin of victory for the Democratic Party, passage of the legislation required all the skills and courage of congressional leaders.

The process involved hard bargaining to fill in gaps in the proposed amendment and to soften its excesses. It involved also maneuvering for support backed by claims for return of past favors. Representative Mills, then chairman of the powerful House Ways and Means Committee, provided the most adroit stroke, which broke the deadlock in the committee and enabled the proposal to be reported out to the floor of the House, where a favorably disposed Congress awaited it. At this time, in early 1965, three bills (four if the AMA's "Eldercare" proposal is included) were still being considered: the administration's hospital insurance bill to be paid through Social Security; the King-Anderson Bill to provide nursing home and home health care, also to be paid for from compulsory contributions to Social Security; and the Byrnes Bill to provide for voluntary health insurance with a federal government subsidy, including in the coverage payment for physicians' services. All three were more or less in competition. Each had its own special purposes, but also its faults. Congressman Mills suggested combining all three into a single package, which with some further compromising finally became the 1965 Amendments to the Social Security Act, providing the legislative basis for Parts A and B of Medicare under Title XVIII. This move made it possible for all parties, except the AMA, to agree that it was a significant achievement; some called it the greatest social innovation since the passage of the original Social Security Act. The final compromise bill passed both houses of Congress and was signed into law by President Johnson in July 1965.

The formulation of a general policy, in summary, reflected the view that the problem of inadequate health services for the elderly was due to their inability to purchase those services. Health care was judged to be a right of all citizens, and not a privilege available only to those who could afford it. Other policy elements that emerged included compulsory insurance, although this was limited to hospital care only, and vendor payments to providers.

This brief statement does not capture either the heat of the argument or the prolonged negotiation that went into the development of the policy statement. It does show that the policy fit only the most narrow definition of the problem. As we shall see, the policy statement also adopted a conventional concept of insurance and accepted the criteria of a model of acute diseases.

Given the background of social values related to health and social insurance in this country, it is not illogical that the primary problem definition should have focused on the economic barriers to health care for the aged, and that a universal, contributory approach should have been conceived as the appropriate policy direction for dealing with their need for assistance in financing this care. From this perspective, it is not surprising that no attempt was made to deal directly with other aspects of the problem of the health and health care needs of the aged. However, various of the policy and program specifics seem scrupulously designed to avoid any suggestion of a purpose other than paying the medical care bills of the aged. The emphasis is so exaggerated that when taken together the specific provisions suggest that effort was directed toward appeasing or co-opting various entities involved in the provision or financing of health care, rather than toward designing a policy and program that would reduce the financial barrier to health care for the aged.

This is illustrated in the first three sections of Title XVIII of the Social

Security Act, which carefully delimit the scope of Medicare. These sections, which appear below in their entirety, constitute an unusual approach in that they specify what the program is not, before there is any discussion of what it is.

Prohibition Against Any Federal Interference

Section 1801. Nothing in this title shall be construed to authorize any Federal officer or employee to exercise any supervision or control over the practice of medicine or the manner in which medical services are provided, or over the selection, tenure, or compensation of any officer or employee of any institution, agency, or person providing health services; or to exercise any supervision or control over the administration or operation of any such institution, agency, or person.

Free Choice by Patient Guaranteed

Section 1802. Any individual entitled to insurance benefits under this title may obtain health services from any institution, agency, or person qualified to participate under this title if such institution, agency, or person undertakes to provide him such services.

Option to Individuals to Obtain Other Health Insurance Protection

Section 1803. Nothing contained in this title shall be construed to preclude any State from providing, or any individual from purchasing or otherwise securing protection against the cost of any health services. (Committee on Finance, United States Senate, 1976, p. 407).

It is stated quite specifically that Medicare will not authorize any interference in the delivery of medical services, the free choice of provider, or the obtaining of other health insurance protection through the state or directly. These specifications protected the interests of providers in having a free hand in the delivery of care, of states in being able to make additional arrangements for care financing that build on Medicare, and of insurance companies in a potentially wider market for health insurance. Medicare was made much more acceptable to insurance companies by installing them as intermediaries between the program and providers.

PROVISIONS OF THE MEDICARE PROGRAM

Recognition of the right to health as a concept was a necessary prerequisite to development of a program that would operationalize this philosophical position, if only for the aged portion of the population. The fact that the legislative process resulting in the Medicare program had its genesis as early as 1912 gives some perspective on how slowly values change. It should be noted that the value changes are reflected in policy and that both the explicit and implicit intentions of policy are put into action in program development. At this point, it is appropriate to describe the Medicare program, technically Title XVIII of the Social Security Act as added by the 1965 amendments.

As originally passed, the Medicare program provides health insurance for people who have reached the age of 65. The 1972 amendments included under the Medicare program workers under age 65 who have been receiving Social Security Disability Insurance benefits for two years or more, and insured persons and their dependents who have end-stage renal disease three months after kidney dialysis begins. Although there are some exceptions, nearly all of the more than 22 million Americans who are 65 years old or older are eligible to receive benefits from this program. There are two different but related parts of the broader program of health insurance: Part A is a hospital insurance plan (HI), which provides protection against the costs of hospital and intermediate institutional care; Part B provides supplementary medical insurance (SMI) as assistance for costs of physician services and certain other ambulatory health services. Part A is automatic; that is, hospital insurance is compulsory for those eligible.

At the inception of the program, enrollment in Part B was established as voluntary and requiring the payment of a monthly premium. Effective July 1979, the premium, which is established annually and can be increased by no more than the percentage increase in general Social Security benefits for the previous year, was $8.70. A major information campaign was launched to inform eligible persons of the advantages of enrolling in this part of the program. The overwhelming majority of the eligible aged enrolled in the program, which indicates its value and appeal. Because of the sustained level of enrollment in Part B, the administrative mechanism was finally reversed, starting in mid-1973, so that persons who establish entitlement to hospital insurance are automatically enrolled in SMI unless they specifically refuse this coverage (Social Security Handbook, 1978).

While the coverage as described seems extensive, it is by no means total. Both Parts A and B involve deductibles and co-insurance for the various benefits. A deductible is the amount of the reasonable charge for a covered service for which the insured individual must take responsibility before Medicare will pay any portion of the bill. Co-insurance is a percentage of the reasonable charge for a covered service the insured individual must pay along with the Medicare payment after any deductible has been satisfied. There is no coverage under Medicare for private nurses, private rooms unless prescribed, prescription drugs except those for use by an in-patient or those that cannot be self-administered, or any form of custodial care. Additionally, personal comfort items for hospital patients, such as telephone or television, are not covered. Part A of Medicare provides hospital insurance benefits but not physicians' services even though received in a hospital. This insurance can help pay for in-patient hospital care if the following four conditions are all met: (1) the hospitalization is prescribed by a physician for treatment of an illness or injury; (2) the kind of care that can be provided only in a hospital is required; (3) the hospital is participating in Medicare (unless treatment is needed for an emergency to prevent death or serious impairment and the nonparticipating hospital is the closest suitable one); and (4) the hospital's Utilization Review Committee or a Professional Standards Review Organization does not disapprove the stay (Your Medicare Handbook, 1976). These benefits are available anew within a "spell of illness," defined as a benefit period beginning with the first day on which an entitled person is furnished with in-patient hospital services and ending after 60 consecutive days thereafter on which she or he was not an in-patient in any hospital or skiled nursing facility. The benefits available within each benefit period include:

1. *Up to 90 days of in-patient hospital care.* Payment is available for board and semiprivate room, regular nursing services, operating room and special care unit charges, drugs administered in the hospital, laboratory texts, x-ray and other radiological services, other medical supplies or appliances furnished by the hospital, and rehabilitation services such as physical therapy. As of 1979, there is a $160 deductible, approximately equal to the cost of the first day of hospitalization, for any covered hospital stay. After the sixtieth day of hospitalization within a "spell of illness," there is a $40 per day co-insurance charge for any of the next 30 days of needed hospital stay. For hospital stays extending beyond 90 days, there is a "lifetime reserve" of 60 days, which is not renewable after it is used. For any of these days that are used, there is a co-insurance charge of $80. In establishing the deductible and co-insurance rates under Part A, a specific relationship was set in law between the respective amounts. The deductible is computed each year using a formula based on the increase in the average per diem rate for in-patient hospital services during the preceding year as compared with 1966. The co-insurance payment for the sixty-first through ninetieth days of hospitalization is equal to one-fourth the deductible. For the ninety-first through one-hundred fiftieth days, the lifetime reserve days, the co-insurance rate is one-half the deductible. The nonrenewable 60 days of reserve available for use once in the individual's lifetime can be used in more than one way. There are two issues of primary concern. One is the possibility that an individual may require an extended period of hospitalization in which the 90 renewable days of in-patient hospital care within a spell of illness are exhausted. This may occur with a terminal illness requiring a long hospitalization. Reserve days might also be used, and less dramatically than in a lengthy terminal hospitalization, when the individual has multiple illness events requiring repeat hospitalization and close enough in time that they are within one spell of illness. As indicated above, a new spell of illness starts only after a 60-day period in which the individual is not an in-patient in any facility. The situation where there is difficulty stabilizing a patient or

where the patient suffers a series of attacks or exacerbations of illness could involve movement from hospital to skilled nursing facility (SNF) to home and through the cycle again several times without a 60 day break so that the spell of illness terminates. This could use up the 90 days of life-time reserve for hospital care without requiring one very long hospital stay. Multiple hospital admissions within the same year are not uncommon among the elderly, particularly among men.

2. *Up to 100 days of posthospital care* in a participating SNF (formerly called ECF or extended are facility). This care is covered by insurance if the individual no longer needs all the services that only a hospital can provide, but still requires daily skilled nursing care or rehabilitation services that can be provided only in a skilled nursing facility. A SNF is a specially qualified facility that has the staff and equipment to provide this care. Hospital insurance cannot pay for the stay if the patient is there mainly because of a need for custodial care, or if the skilled nursing or rehabilitation services are needed only occasionally (for example, once or twice a week). All of the following five conditions have to be met if the insurance is to help pay for the care: (a) the individual has been in a hospital at least three consecutive days not counting the day of discharge; (b) the patient was transferred to the SNF because the condition treated in the hospital requires care; (c) the patient is admitted to the facility within a short time (generally 14 days) after leaving the hospital; (d) a physician certifies the need for skilled nursing or skilled rehabilitation services on a daily basis, and these are actually received; and, (5) the SNF's Utilization Review Committee or a Professional Standards Review Organization does not disapprove the stay (Your Medicare Handbook, 1976). Payment is provided for board and semiprivate room, special modalities of therapy, and other services similar to those available in a hospital, such as regular nursing services and drugs. There is a co-insurance charge of $18 per day (beginning in 1978) for SNF stays after the first 20 days.

3. *Up to 100 home health service visits* in the year following discharge from a hospital or SNF after the beginning of one benefit period and before the start of the next. Medicare can help pay for skilled health services needed only on a part-time basis by persons confined to their homes because of an illness or injury. Both Part A and Part B provide benefits for home care, but for Part A coverage, the individual must have been an in-patient in a hospital or skilled nursing facility. However, Medicare does not cover this care if it is furnished primarily to assist people in meeting personal, family, and domestic needs. Payment is provided for part-time skilled nursing care, and physical and speech therapy. Payment can be provided for any of the following if they are needed: occupational therapy, part-time services of home health aids, medical social services, and medical supplies and equipment furnished by the agency. There are no deductible or co-insurance charges for covered services for these 100 visits. All of the following six

conditions must be met if hospital insurance is to pay for home health visits: (a) the patient was in a hospital for at least three consecutive days not counting the day of discharge; (b) the care is for further treatment of a condition treated in a hospital or skilled nursing facility; (c) the care needed includes part-time skilled nursing care, physical therapy, or speech therapy; (d) the patient is confined to home; (e) a physician determines the need for home health care and sets up a plan within 14 days after the patient's discharge from a hospital or participating skilled nursing facility; and (f) the home health agency is participating in Medicare (Your Medicare Handbook, 1976).

Payments for physicians' services, which are conspicuously absent from the benefits of Part A, are the principal benefit under Part B, the voluntary medical insurance part of the program. Partial financial support is provided for medical and surgical services of doctors of medicine and osteopathy, and for dental surgery. This does not include ordinary dental care, but does include charges for diagnostic tests and procedures, medical supplies, and certain drugs administered by the physician. Under certain conditions these benefits can be obtained by an out-patient in a hospital clinic or by a patient in a physician's private office. Omitted from coverage under either Part A or Part B are preventive health services (such as routine physical examinations or immunizations), eyeglasses, hearing aids, and any form of custodial care. In general, there is a 20 percent co-insurance payment required of the reasonable charge for all covered services above the deductible under Part B. The yearly deductible was set at $50 at the start of the program, subject to periodic review. As of January 1, 1973 it was $60. Payment for home health service visits is available under Part B subject to the deductible, but not a co-insurance charge, provided the following four conditions are all met: (1) part-time skilled nursing care or physical or speech therapy is needed; (2) a physician determines the need for services and sets up a plan for home health care; (3) the patient is confined to home; and (4) the home health agency is participating in Medicare (Your Medicare Handbook, 1976).

Help is available to pay for blood under both Parts A and B of Medicare, except for the first three pints, for which the individual is responsible. Under Part A, the full cost of additional blood is paid for an in-patient in a hospital or a skilled nursing facility. Under Part B, additional blood received as an out-patient or as part of other covered services can be paid for subject to deductible and co-insurance provisions on the reasonable charge.

The concept mentioned several times above of reasonable or "usual, customary, and reasonable" (UCR) charge is important in determining acceptable fees under the program. Reasonable charges vary from one region of the country to another and generally reflect differences in the cost of living. Under both Part A (hospital insurance) and Part B (supplementary medical insurance) of Medicare, the payment for covered services provided to beneficiaries by hospitals, skilled nursing facilities, and home health agencies is based on either the reasonable cost for providing the services or the customary charges for these services, whichever is less. The lesser of the two is used as the basis for health benefit payments to these facilities. Reasonable costs are computed on various bases. Regardless of the method used, the objective is to approximate as closely as practicable the actual direct and indirect cost of services provided to beneficiaries. The intent is that the cost of services to individuals covered under Medicare not be borne by those who are not covered, and, similarly, that the cost of services to persons who are not covered not be borne by Medicare.

The secretary of Health, Education, and Welfare is authorized to limit accepted provider costs based on the comparable costs of services of various classes of providers in the same area (Social Security Handbook, 1978). Under Part B (SMI), the usual, customary, and reasonable fee charged for a service is the basis for paying for a physician's services or for medical and other health services furnished by nonphysician parties that are not hospitals, skilled nursing facilities, or home health agencies. The medical insurance carrier serving as intermediary assures that the charges are not higher than those to the carrier's own policyholders for comparable services or than what is usually charged for similar services. Additionally, the prevailing charges in the locality for similar services are used as a standard of an acceptable fee. The prevailing charge limit in a locality is calculated on the seventy-fifth percentile of the customary charges for physicians or others who provide that service*—for example, a routine office visit or a diagnostic x-ray (Social Security Handbook, 1978). In essence, this sets the seventy-fifth percentile of the distribution of physician charges for a service in the locality served by an insurance carrier as the highest acceptable fee. The individual is responsible for the deductible and co-insurance amounts using this fee level as the highest base. Any amount a physician charges above this seventy-fifth percentile is considered in excess of the usual, customary, and reasonable charge for that service and is not the responsibility of the Medicare program but of the patient. Under most circumstances, physicians may charge whatever they wish for a service, regardless of whether Medicare or any private insurance mechanism will honor the total bill. In other words, the policy of UCR limits the reimbursement, but not the cost of health care, thus seriously affecting the objective of Medicare, which is to reduce the financial barriers to adequate health care.

If a physician has agreed to accept an assignment of benefits due a patient, then the reasonable charge must be accepted as the full charge. Under this arrangement, payment is made directly to the physician after the

---

*Increases to the prevailing charge levels are permitted subject to the economic index limitation only to the extent that the increases are determined to be justified by the secretary of Health, Education, and Welfare based on appropriate data.

reasonable charge has been reduced by any unmet deductible and the 20 percent co-insurance amount. The physician agrees not to charge the patient an amount in excess of any unmet deductible and 20 percent of the reasonable charges (Social Security Handbook, 1978). The patient is responsible for paying the deductible and co-insurance amounts directly or through some other public or private health insurance mechanism. When assignment has not been arranged, the individual pays physicians' bills and is reimbursed after the deductible has been met and the co-insurance amount subtracted.

The Medicaid program provides another source of payment for the medical care needs of an individual age 65 and over. However, as discussed earlier, eligibility for this program requires an aged person to establish financial need for this assistance. For persons eligible for both Medicare and Medicaid, it is in a state's best interest to transfer as much as possible of the cost of health care to the Medicare program. Medicare is federally financed; Medicaid is jointly financed by the state and Federal government. The state government may be responsible for as much as 50 percent of the cost of the Medicaid program, with such an equal sharing a common arrangement.

One mechanism states can use to transfer costs to the Medicare program is to buy coverage under Part B (SMI) for persons eligible to enroll in the program who are receiving Medicaid. This option is available to a state if it has entered into an agreement to do so with the secretary of Health, Education, and Welfare before the start of 1970. When this has been done, the deductibles and co-insurance applicable under Medicare and the Part B premium are paid by Medicaid, and the remainder of the reasonable costs and charges of covered services are paid by Medicare.

PROBLEM, POLICY, AND PROGRAM: THE CASE OF THE IMPERFECT FIT

The Medicare program represents the results of more than 50 years of legislative bargaining, lobbying and counterlobbying, pressure, pleading, and politics. It is a compromise between the forces that wanted no part of such a program and proponents who wanted much more. As such, it reflects both explicit and implicit goals of the legislation. The *explicit* intent, of course, was to provide financial assistance to the elderly for medical services; that is, to reduce, but not eliminate, the financial barrier to obtaining needed medical care. The *implicit* intent was more subtle and more far-reaching: to develop a system of comprehensive health services in American communities by encouraging voluntary cooperation among the health service providers—physicians and other health personnel, hospitals, nursing homes, and home health agencies (Congressional Record cvii, March 5, 1962, 3112–13). Initially, it was estimated that existing community health resources would be inadequate to meet the anticipated steep rise in demand for services. Lack of resources, coupled with already rising costs of care, led policy makers to expect Medicare could be used to stimulate development of alternatives to crisis-oriented, acute care that would be more appropriate to the actual health needs of the elderly. Thus, reimbursement policy and procedures, among other elements, were designed to encourage collaboration among providers of health services to the elderly, as a way of reducing other barriers to care, such as availability and accessibility.

Our general hypothesis is that there is an "imperfect fit" between the underlying dimensions of the problem, the intent of the policy, and the operationalization of that intent in the Medicare program. In other words, we hypothesize that Medicare, despite some positive achievements, is an inadequate program solution to the problem addressed by the policy. Given the definition of the problem as described above, the highest priority of the Medicare program was to relieve the burden of health care costs and reduce the then-existing relationship between utilization of health services and income status.

As we have stated elsewhere,

> Some aspects of the program were intended to stimulate or reinforce development of services and facilities considered medically necessary or potentially less costly, e.g., home health services and extended care facilities. However, there was no explicit intent to alter the traditional system of fee-for-service medicine. The program provided a guarantee of payment for certain hospital and medical services to a population group which previously could not always pay its medical bills. As such, the program could have been considered a support for the existing medical care system with little incentive for provision of more effective medical care for the aged population. Nevertheless, there was an implicit intent to use this mechanism to improve the distribution of needed services to the aged to upgrade the quality of medical care available to this population group by stimulating development of intermediate levels of care, improving access to services, and encouraging cooperation among various providers in the community (Coe, Brehm, and Peterson, 1974).

We have already commented that the policy that resulted in Medicare focused on too narrow a definition of the problem of the health and health care needs of the aged. In this sense, we suggest there was a mismatch between the problem and the policy formulated to deal with it. Health and health care in its interaction with other life circumstances in elderly families is not one problem, but rather a complex combination of several. This complexity was not considered in the definition that led to Medicare.

It is within this context that the impact of Medicare will be assessed. The degree to which Medicare met both its explicit and implicit expectations and goals and the implications of the fit between program specifics and policy intent in this process are the subject of the next chapters.

4

MEDICARE AND THE DELIVERY, USE, AND COST OF HEALTH SERVICES

INTRODUCTION

The analytic model we are using of the match among problem, policy, and program directs our attention to specific aspects of the relationship between Medicare and the health status and health care of the aged. We have already noted the restricted policy focus based on a narrow problem definition. As a result, no direct program effect would be expected on any dimension of the problem except that dimension related to the burden of medical care costs among the aged. Given the assumption that an increased ability to pay for medical care services would stimulate the development or expansion of those service mechanisms most appropriate to the needs of the elderly, an indirect effect would be expected on a variety of medical care organization and delivery considerations. Our hypothesis that there was also an imperfect fit between the program and the policy it was intended to implement leads us to anticipate, based on program design features, performance shortcomings even at the level of dealing with the burden of medical care costs among the aged.

Essentially, three areas of concern related to the impact of Medicare on the delivery, use, and cost of medical care services stem from our hypothesis. These are: (1) the impact on affordability, as the explicit intent of the policy and program; (2) the impact on promotion of availability of services appropriate to the health needs of the elderly, which was the implicit intent and (3) the impact on coordination of health services for the aged. This last item can be regarded as implicit in the general intent to encourage effective and efficient use and delivery of care so as to limit unnecessary program expenditures.

In reviewing the impact on affordability, we will consider utilization, before and after Medicare was implemented, of basic health services such as physician services and hospital care as well as the changes in overall costs and the amount of these costs borne by the aged. Our concern for availability focuses on the development and expansion of health services most relevant to the special health needs of the elderly; that is, services oriented to illness management for the chronic diseases, as contrasted to acute care. Of particular interest is the impact of Medicare on the availability of a range and levels of treatment modalities that might work to control the overall costs of care while at the same time providing more appropriate mechanisms of care. These include home health care services that might shorten or avoid a hospital stay and intermediate care facilities (skilled nursing facilities).

The concern for the coordination among health care delivery organizations and providers is related to the impact of Medicare on the development of more effective working relationships among elements in the health care system directed toward delivery of comprehensive care. This includes such issues as transfer and referral to appropriate levels of care and the orientation of providers toward caring for the chronic diseases. Since the program presumably guarantees payments, as a basic right, a primary consideration in reviewing the impact of Medicare on organizational relationships is the way in which the coverage and reimbursement policies of the insurance program itself might have influenced these relationships.

AFFORDABILITY

Some areas of public income maintenance, social programs, and service delivery are oriented primarily towards the needs of the aged. However, health services in this country are not aimed principally at meeting their demands. All segments of the population make demands on the existing health care delivery resources, although unquestionably these demands vary in amount and kind. In attempting to review the effects of Medicare on the use and cost of different types of health services among the aged, we will look at changing patterns over time for the aged, with other age groups serving as a basis for comparison. Of particular concern is how this change relates to the original intent of the program and the situation that existed around the time the program was being considered. We will also consider the relationship of Medicare to the differential patterns of use of care by older women as compared with older men and how use patterns have changed differently for major categories of care and by sex.

As indicated in Chapter 3, a person age 65 or over who is entitled to receive a Social Security monthly cash benefit, whether or not receiving it, is provided protection under Part A of Medicare; virtually all persons who became 65 before 1968 were brought into Medicare regardless of eligibility for other benefits. Persons 65 or over can be eligible for Medicare based on their own or their spouse's work in employment covered for Social

Security purposes. However, unlike retirement, survivors, and disability benefits, the payment of benefits under the Medicare program is not differentially based on the prior earnings of the individual. Any differences in benefits paid are due to the then-prevailing patterns of use of care, the costs of different services used, and characteristics of the design of the Medicare program. (These design characteristics are the services covered and the way in which deductibles and co-insurance are applied.) Similarly, changes in the patterns of use and cost of services over time may have been caused when these design characteristics reinforced emphasized certain patterns of use, with a resultant impact on the cost of these services. This may also have differentially affected different segments of the elderly population.

The Medicare reimbursement approach was designed principally to pay hospital expenses for short-stay hospital care (Gibson and Fisher, 1979), thus relieving the aged of the potentially major financial burden of such care. As is still true, the most expensive form of medical care services when the program was first initiated was in-patient hospital care. This was despite the fact that data from the 1963 Social Security Survey of the Aged (Epstein and Murray, 1967) indicated both married couples and nonmarried women who incurred medical costs had higher percentages of their mean cost of all care for physician and surgeon services and medications than for expenses at hospitals and other medical institutions.

In 1967, the first full year of Medicare's operations, in-patient hospital services accounted for 63 percent of the total Medicare bill, while physician and other medical services were 29 percent of the bill. By 1976 the emphasis on hospital care had increased to the point where in-patient hospital services were 70 percent of the program bill and physician services 23 percent. If the Medicare program had been oriented toward stimulating use of ambulatory care alternatives to in-patient hospital care where this was appropriate, it might have served the dual objective of promoting the use of the least expensive form of care suitable in a given situation at the same time that it reduced the financial barrier to obtaining needed care. The actual experience since Medicare began does not reflect such a situation.

Physician Visits

As Table 4.1 shows, there were 4.8 physician visits per person per year for all age groups in 1977. For those 65 and over, the rate was 6.5. For those 45 and over, the differences among age groups in the number of visits have, if anything, become smaller since 1963. For the total population, there has been an irregular pattern with an overall small increase in average visits per year since shortly after Medicare began. However, the first years of Medicare showed a small drop in the average number of visits from the 1963–64 period. For those 65–74, the pattern is similar but somewhat more stable.

TABLE 4.1: Number of Physician Visits per Person per Year, 1963–77

	July 1963–June 1964	July 1966–June 1967	1969	1971	1973	1975	1977
All persons	4.5	4.3	4.3	4.9	5.0	5.1	4.8
Age:							
Under 5 years	5.5	5.7	5.7	6.8	6.5	6.9	4.1[a]
5–14	2.8	2.7	2.8	3.3	3.4	3.4	
15–24	4.3	4.0	3.7	4.5	4.5	4.4	4.3[b]
25–34	4.7	4.4	4.4	5.1	5.3	5.2	4.7
35–44	4.4	4.3	4.1	4.5	4.9	4.8	
45–54	4.8	4.3	4.3	5.1	5.4	5.4	5.4
55–64	5.3	5.1	5.1	5.9	5.5	5.9	
65–74	6.3	6.0	6.1	6.4	6.5	6.6	6.6
75 and over	7.3	6.0	6.2	7.2	6.6	6.6	6.5

[a] Under 17 years.
[b] 17–24 years.

Source: National Center for Health Statistics, Series 10, No. 97, 1975 (Table B); Series 10, No. 128, 1979 (Table 7); and Series 10, No. 126, 1978 (Table 20).

There was a drop in average number of physician visits per person per year in the first few years of Medicare, and then an increase in 1971 to slightly above the pre-Medicare level. The rate has been basically the same since then. For those 75 and over, there is an irregular pattern that shows a sizable drop in average number of visits from before to the first years after Medicare. The rate increase in 1971 to almost what it was pre-Medicare, and then dropped off again. It has been virtually unchanged since, and additionally has shown no difference compared with the rate for those 65–74. The rate of physician visits per person per year in 1977 was lower for those 75 and over than it was before Medicare started; for those 65–74 it was only slightly higher.

The Medicare program data in Table 4.2 show the changes from 1967 to 1976 in the use and cost of physician and other medical services under SMI. There were 359 persons served per 1,000 enrollees in 1967. The figure increased to 546 per 1,000 in 1976, a 52 percent increase. However, it is not possible to compare this directly to the NCHS data just discussed, for various reasons. Of major importance is that the program measure of persons served per 1,000 enrolled is directly affected by increased charges for physician services. These increased charges cause more people to meet the Part B deductible, with no necessary increase in the use of physician services. The annual Part B deductible has increased by only $10 since the program started. Additionally, average visits per person is a measure of extent of use, whereas persons served per 1,000 enrolled is a measure of use-nonuse, even considering the effect of the deductible. While maintaining the deductible with only a relatively minor increase could have been a spur to greater actual physician use, this does not seem to have been the case. Possibly this is so because the co-insurance rate is unchanged and this still requires a major share of the cost of physician visits to be borne out-of-pocket by the aged individual.

The total reimbursement for physician and other medical services under the program increased from 1967 to 1976 from $1.2 billion to $3.6 billion, or by 197 percent. On an individual basis, the reimbursement per person served increased from $191 to $297, or by 56 percent, during the same period. The reimbursement per person enrolled increased by 137 percent, from $68 to $162. The increased reimbursement per person served reflects primarily changes in the unit cost of services provided to users and the increase in average number of physician visits since the early years of Medicare. The rate of increase from 1967 to 1976 in the reimbursement per person enrolled is much greater because this measure, like persons served per 1,000 enrolled, is affected by the increased number of individuals obtaining reimbursement because unit cost increases caused more persons to satisfy the deductible.

The implications of these various increases in physician use under Medicare from the first full calendar year of program operations until the last year for which data are available will become more apparent when we

**TABLE 4.2:   Use of Physician and Other Medical Services under
SMI for Persons 65 and over, 1967 and 1976**

Usage Indicator	1967	1976	Percent Change 1967-76
Persons served per 1,000 enrolled			
Total	358.5	545.5	+52.2
Male	345.6	520.9	+50.7
Female	368.0	562.0	+52.7
Reimbursement total (in $1,000)			
Total	$1,223,845	$3,632,539	+196.8
Male	551,418	1,573,363	+185.3
Female	672,428	2,059,177	+206.2
Reimbursement per person served			
Total	$190.77	$296.69	+55.5
Male	211.41	333.84	+57.9
Female	176.62	273.44	+54.8
Reimbursement per person enrolled			
Total	$68.40	$161.84	+136.6
Male	73.07	173.91	+138.1
Female	64.99	153.68	+136.5

Source: U.S. Department of Health, Education, and Welfare, Medicare 1967 and Medicare 1975-76.

compare this information with data on the use of other services under the
program and analyze the differences by sex.

Hospital Care

There are more pronounced differences over time in the use of in-
patient hospital services, as seen in NCHS and program data. As Tables 4.3
and 4.4 show, the rate of admission to short-term general hospitals has
grown substantially over the years for the population 65 and over, particularly from before to after the introduction of Medicare. It was 275 per 1,000
persons in 1967, rising to 314 per 1,000 in 1971 (in 1964 65 the discharge rate
had been 183 per 1,000.* The data on the population 65 and over enrolled in
Medicare show the same trends. In 1969, the hospital admission rate was 307

---

*Some data report hospital utilization in admission rates, others in discharge rates.
Admission rates are consistently higher than discharge rates.

TABLE 4.3: Short-Term General Hospital Utilization for Persons 65 and over

Indicator	1967	1968	1969	1970	1971
Admission rate per 1,000 persons 65 and over	275	285	301	310	314
Average length of stay (days)	12.7	13.3	13.2	12.8	12.4

Source: West (1971).

per 1,000 enrollees, rising to 320 per 1,000 in 1973. However, whether admission or discharge data are used, the trend over time is the same. More recent NCHS data for 1975 (admissions) and 1977 (discharges) reflect a continuing increase in the use of short-stay in-patient hospital facilities.

While hospital admission and discharge rates have been increasing, average lengths of stay have been generally decreasing for the aged, after an upswing during the first few years after Medicare was implemented. This may represent an increase in the use of in-patient care for less serious illnesses. The balance between these two measures has resulted in relative stability in days of care per 1,000 after an initial upswing, so that there is almost no difference in days of care per 1,000 for 1967 and 1973.

The Medicare program data in Table 4.5 show the changes from 1967 to 1976 in the use and cost of in-patient hospital services under HI. The average number of persons served per 1,000 enrolled increased from 185 to 227 between 1967 and 1976. This 23 percent increase reflects an actual increase in the number of persons using in-patient hospital services. Unlike the situation for SMI, there is no basis for assuming that any of the change in average number of persons served per 1,000 enrolled is the result of a change in the number of people meeting the HI deductible. This deductible has maintained a more consistent relationship over the course of the program to the approximate cost of the first day of hospitalization than the SMI deductible has to the cost of a physician visit.

TABLE 4.4: All Hospital In-patient Admissions of Hospital Insurance Enrollees under Medicare

Indicator	1969	1970	1971	1972	1973
Admission rate per 1,000 HI enrollees	307	307	305	313	320
Average length of covered stay (days)	—	13.1	12.6	12.1	11.7

Source: U.S. Department of Health, Education, and Welfare (1976b).
—=not available.

TABLE 4.5:   Use of In-patient Hospital Services under HI for Persons 65 and over, 1967 and 1976

Usage Indicator	1967	1976	Percent Change, 1967–76
Persons served per 1,000 enrolled			
Total	184.7	227.4	+23.1
Male	198.3	241.5	+21.8
Female	174.8	217.7	+24.5
Reimbursement total (in $1,000)			
Total	$2,659,393	$10,979,662	+312.9
Male	1,233,979	4,842,710	+292.4
Female	1,425,414	6,136,952	+330.5
Reimbursement per person served			
Total	$738.46	$2,106.70	+185.3
Male	755.07	2,150.31	+184.8
Female	724.66	2,073.52	+186.1
Reimbursement per person enrolled			
Total	$136.42	$479.03	+251.1
Male	149.70	519.38	+246.9
Female	126.69	451.36	+256.3

Source: U.S. Department of Health, Education, and Welfare, *Medicare 1967* and *Medicare 1975–76.*

The total reimbursement for in-patient hospital services under HI increased from just over $2.5 billion to almost $11 billion between 1967 and 1976, a 313 percent increase. Reimbursement per person served increased by 185 percent to $2,106.70, and reimbursement per person enrolled increased by 251 percent to $479.03. The pattern of these increases shows the effect of both increased unit costs and increased rates of use for in-patient hospital services. Total reimbursement and reimbursement per person enrolled are affected by both these factors and show the highest rates of increase.

The rates of increase for use of and reimbursement for services under the program have been much greater for in-patient care than for physician and other medical services, except for average number of persons served per 1,000 enrolled. However, as explained above, this measure is directly affected by the number of persons meeting the SMI deductible, and the percentage increase does not reflect an actual increase in the use of physician services. The absolute numbers of dollars involved in total and per-person reimbursement are obviously many times higher for in-patient hospital services than for physician services, and have grown at a much more substantial rate.

These changes in relative use of hospital, as compared with physician, services have implications for the overall increases in program expenditures. There are differences between the sexes in patterns of use of these services that bear on the changes in use and reimbursements during Medicare's first decade.

Differences by Sex

In 1963, two years before the Medicare amendments passed, 56 percent of the population 65 and over was female, and the ratio of females to males has increased since. In 1966, 57 percent of Medicare enrollees were female; in 1975, 59 percent were female. The largest single category of older women was widows in 1963, with just over half of all older women in this group.

The median income of all nonmarried women, the largest category of all older people, was about 30 percent less than the median income of the much smaller group of nonmarried men, and about one-third the income of married couples with at least one member 65 and over.

According to the medical care use data from the 1963 Social Security Survey of the Aged, men had more short-stay hospital discharges per 1,000 persons than did women, because of a higher frequency of multiple hospitalizations, while women had more physician visits. Direct comparisons by sex were not available for this study, but nonmarried women had somewhat higher total medical care costs and out-of-pocket costs than did men.

At the time Medicare was passed, the group in greatest economic need, as well as the largest group among the aged, was nonmarried women. They tended to use ambulatory care relatively more often and hospital in-patient care relatively less often than men.

The data in Table 4.6 show that, as of 1967, there were 21.5 discharges from short-stay hospitals per 100 men and 18.3 discharges per 100 women

TABLE 4.6: Short-Stay Hospital Discharges per 100 Persons per Year, by Sex, for Persons Age 65 and over

Year	Total	Male	Female
1963–64	19.0	19.5	18.6
1967	19.7	21.5	18.3
1970	23.4	25.3	22.0
1974	25.4	28.1	23.5
1977	27.5	30.3	25.4

Source: National Center for Health Statistics, *Utilization of Short-Stay Hospitals, 1979.*

age 65 and over. There was an overall increase in this rate from 1963–64 based on the rate increase for men. There was no increased use for women until 1970. Medicare statistics similarly showed more older men than women per 1,000 enrolled served for in-patient hospital care. While total reimbursements for such care were higher for women than for men, this was the result of a larger number of women than men in this age group. The per-person-served and per-person-enrolled reimbursement rates were higher for men than for women. This is not unexpected, given the higher rates of use of in-patient care by older men.

The 1966–67 data in Table 4.7 on physician visits per year, from the National Health Survey, show more visits per person for women than for men in both the 65–74 and the 75-and-over age categories. Medicare statistics for 1967 similarly show more older women per 1,000 enrolled served than men for physician and other medical service. The total reimbursement was also higher for women than for men for such care. However, the per-person-served and the per-person-enrolled reimbursements were higher for men than for women despite a higher per-person number of physician visits among older women.

TABLE 4.7: Physician Visits per Person per Year, by Sex, for Persons Age 65–74 and 75 and over

Year	Total	Male	Female
1966–67			
65–74	6.0	5.6	6.3
75 and over	6.0	5.1	6.7
1970			
65–74	6.0	5.7	6.2
75 and over	6.7	6.2	7.1
1971			
65–74	6.4	6.0	6.7
75 and over	7.2	6.5	7.6
1974			
65–74	6.9	6.8	6.9
75 and over	6.5	6.3	6.6
1975			
65–74	6.6	6.3	6.8
75 and over	6.6	6.5	6.7
1977			
65–74	6.5	6.4	6.6
75 and over	6.5	6.4	6.6

Source: National Center for Health Statistics, Volume of physician visits, 1979.

The figures in Table 4.8 for overall use and reimbursement under both parts of Medicare for 1967 indicate that more women than men were enrolled, that more women than men per 1,000 enrolled were served, and that more money was spent in total on women than on men, but that reimbursement per person served and per person enrolled was higher for men than for women.

When we move forward in time and review data for the 1976–77 period, we see some interesting patterns. Between 1967 and 1977, according to the National Health Survey data, there was a 40 percent increase for both sexes in the short-stay hospital discharge rates. Medicare statistics showed the

TABLE 4.8: Use of HI and/or SMI for Persons 65 and over, 1967 and 1976

Usage Indicator	1967	1976	Percent Change 1967–76
Ever enrolled			
Total	20,715,546	24,624,539	+18.9
Male	8,843,568	10,076,628	+13.9
Female	11,871,978	14,547,911	+22.5
Persons served per 1,000 enrolled			
Total	366.5	554.6	+51.3
Male	357.1	531.1	+48.7
Female	373.4	570.6	+52.8
Reimbursement total (in $1,000)			
Total	$4,238,633	$15,679,687	+269.9
Male	1,907,689	6,819,200	+257.4
Female	2,330,944	8,860,467	+280.1
Reimbursement per person served			
Total	$592.45	$1,214.96	+105.1
Male	646.83	1,361.49	+110.4
Female	554.31	1,122.02	+102.4
Reimbursement per person enrolled			
Total	$217.13	—*	—
Male	230.99	—	—
Female	206.97	—	—

*Data not available.

Source: U.S. Department of Health, Education, and Welfare, Medicare 1967 and Medicare 1975–76.

same pattern in 1976 as in 1967. There was a higher number of males served per 1,000 enrollees, and the reimbursement per person served and per person enrolled was higher for men.

The National Health Survey data on physician visits per person per year do not show as marked an increase from 1967 to 1977 as do the data on hospital discharges. There is, however, a more definite pattern of increase for older men than for older women. For women there is minor change in the physician visit rate over the decade. For men the rate per person per year increased for those 65–74 by 14 percent over the decade, and for those 75 and over by 26 percent. For women, the rate increased by 5 percent for those 65–74 and actually dropped by 1 to 2 percent for those 75 and over. As this difference in pattern suggests, the physician visits per person per year rates for men and women were much closer to each other in 1977 than in 1967. However, women did show a consistently higher rate of physician visits over the time period.

When we look at the overall Medicare statistics in Table 4.8, we find that between 1967 and 1976 there was a 270 percent increase in total annual reimbursement, from $4.2 billion to $15.7 billion. The reimbursement per person served increased by 105 percent, with a slightly higher rate of increase for men than for women. Men continued to show a higher level of reimbursement per person served than women.

For in-patient hospital services, the 1976 data continue to show higher rates of persons served per 1,000 enrolled for men than for women, and higher reimbursement per person served and per person enrolled. However, the rates of increase from 1967 to 1976 are consistently if only slightly higher for women than for men on all these measures, possibly suggesting a slight narrowing of the gap.

For physician and other medical services, the 1976 data again show more women than men served per 1,000 enrolled, but higher levels of reimbursement per person served and per person enrolled for men than for women. Older men may use physician services less frequently than older women, but they presumably use more expensive services.

When we compare the rates of increase from 1967 to 1976 in levels of reimbursement for in-patient hospital services and physician and other medical services, we can see the potential effect of program characteristics on the use and cost of medical services as this interacts with the different patterns of use between the sexes. The rates of change were basically similar for both sexes, but not for the two major categories of care. These presumed effects of Medicare demonstrate the degree to which patterns and trends in medical care use may be alterable based on the introduction of a financing system or a change in the system available.

Persons served per 1,000 enrollees increased from 1967–76 for physician and other medical services by 51 percent for men and 53 percent for women. As discussed previously, this increase was probably based on higher physician charges in 1976 compared with 1967, causing more older persons to meet the deductible. As the National Health Survey data indicated, physician visits per person per year did not show a substantial increase in the period. Persons served per 1,000 enrollees increased for in-patient hospital services by 22 percent for men and 25 percent for women, reflecting an actual increase in use of these services.

Total reimbursement for physician and other services increased by 185 percent for men and 206 percent for women. For in-patient hospital services, the figures were 292 percent and 331 percent, respectively. The higher rates of increase on this measure for women than for men are related to increases in the relative size of the female population among the elderly.

Reimbursement per person served increased for physician and other medical services by 58 percent for men and 55 percent for women. For in-patient hospital services, the increases from 1967 to 1976 were 185 percent for men and 186 percent for women. Reimbursement per person enrolled increased for physician and other services by 138 percent for men and 137 percent for women. For in-patient hospital services, the increases were 247 percent for men and 256 percent for women. These figures represent substantially greater levels of increase for in-patient hospital services than for physician and other medical services. Not only have Medicare reimbursement levels been higher on a per-person basis for older men than for older women since the program started, but the tendency since the program's inception has been for the most rapid increases to be for the most expensive form of care, in-patient hospital services.

It is apparent that the design of the program's reimbursement methods, oriented principally toward paying hospital expenses, encouraged the use of in-patient hospital care rather than ambulatory care services. The program has accommodated more the pre-Medicare male pattern than the female pattern of medical care use. However, while older women make somewhat greater relative use of ambulatory care services than do older men, they also have shown large increases since Medicare in their use of in-patient hospital services. Efforts to alter the patterns of use of health services to increase ambulatory and reduce in-patient care are relevant to older women as much as to older men.

Unequal Use of Benefits

The differences in use patterns by sex point out some implications of the program designed to implement the policy of reducing the financial barriers to health care for the aged. Davis's (1975) examination of data on the distribution of program benefits by socioeconomic characteristics revealed that these benefits were not being equally distributed. In a penetrating analysis using 1968 program data, she demonstrated that the explicit intent of providing equal access for all elderly to needed medical care through lowering financial barriers was not being fulfilled. In terms of income level, race, and availability of services, the program seened to be benefiting most those who had the least need.

The issue of disparity between the races in use of Medicare services was re-examined for the period between 1967 and 1976 (Ruther, 1979). It was found that the initial disparity between aged whites and minorities in persons served per 1,000 enrolled for the overall program declined between 1967 and 1976 from 44 percent (higher for whites) to 13 percent higher. For in-patient care under HI, the difference between the races fell from 36 percent (higher for whites) in 1967 to 19 percent higher in 1976. For physician and other medical services under SMI, there was a 49 percent higher number of persons served per 1,000 for whites in 1967; by 1976 the difference fell to 16 percent. Most of the declines took place in the earlier years of the period analyzed.

The greatest difference by race in use of any service was for skilled nursing facilities. The user rate for whites was 2.8 times higher than that for minorities in 1967. As of 1976, it was 1.7 times higher (Ruther, 1979). During this period, the rate dropped for whites and stayed relatively stable for minority group members. Use of these services for all races has been at a relatively low level.

For out-patient care, minorities consistently had a higher user rate, although this diminished somewhat between 1967 and 1976. On the other hand, home health care under both HI and SMI showed the lowest differentials between white and minority user rates in 1967 (except for out-patient services). For both categories of home health care, user rates were higher for minorities than whites by 1976.

The differences by race in the reimbursement per person served have not been large at any point. However, it shifted for total Medicare services from 6 percent higher for whites in 1967 to 3 percent higher for minorities in 1976. There was a difference in 1976 between in-patient hospital services and physician and other medical services in which group received more reimbursement. In both cases, the movement between 1967 and 1976 was in favor of larger relative reimbursement for minority group members, but this was much less the case for physician services. In 1976, there was a higher level of reimbursement per person served for in-patient hospital care for aged minority-group members than for aged whites. For physician services the drop from 1967 to 1976 was small.

Reimbursement per person enrolled, which combines the effect of user rate and reimbursement per person served, was 53 percent higher overall for whites in 1967, but only 10 percent higher by 1976. The disparity in 1976 was greater for physician services (32 percent) than for in-patient care (5 percent). These data suggest that over time Medicare removed but did not eliminate the gap between the races in the user rate for covered services, especially in the use of ambulatory care services rather than in-patient care.

For reimbursement under the program, the disparity per person served was not great in the early days of the program and actually shifted, except for physician services, to favor minority groups, the most economically depressed. The disparity between the races in reimbursement per person enrolled also narrowed over time, but in this case more for in-patient care than for physician services.

The Cost of Health Care for the Aged

Given the economic circumstances of the elderly, one of the major issues underlying Medicare's development, the relief from out-of-pocket expenses for medical services afforded by the program, is a prime concern. The elderly perceive that problems still exist in meeting the cost of care. The data support the accuracy of these perceptions, in that out-of-pocket costs of care are highest for the elderly in terms of proportion of income.

In 1975, the aged paid more for their health care than they did before Medicare went into effect. This reflects the dramatic increase in total spending for health care from before to after Medicare. Despite a declining share of total expenditures, the absolute amount of his or her own dollars each elderly person spent was greater. Direct out-of-pocket payments for services came to 29 percent of the fiscal year 1975 per-person bill, or $390.00, compared with 53 percent, or $237, in fiscal year 1966. The estimated total direct out-of-pocket payment for health care, including SMI premiums, was 22–24 percent of the average Social Security retired worker's cash benefit in 1975. In fiscal year 1966, just before the start of Medicare, direct payments, including health insurance premiums, came to an estimated 30–32 percent of the average Social Security cash benefit (Gornick, 1976). While this represents a definite decrease in relative level of use of limited resources for direct health care payment by the aged, a relative reduction of about 25 percent in the level of out-of-pocket expenses, it hardly reflects for them a major release from the burdens of financing care.

The trends noted in the use of physicians and hospitals, in combination with inflation rates, have significantly affected the overall and the per capita levels of expenditures for health care and the percentage of the gross national product used for health-related goods and services over the last several years. Data on national health expenditures and the changes that took place from 1965 to 1976 are revealing (Gibson and Mueller, 1976). The total national health expenditure in fiscal year 1966 was $39 billion, which amounted to 5.9 percent of the gross national product. Preliminary estimates for fiscal year 1976 show a total expenditure of $139 billion, or 8.6 percent of the gross national product. The per capita expenditure rose in the same time period from $197.75 to $637.97. Most of the increase in total expenditure is the result of inflation in unit costs and increases in levels of utilization.

When we look at the change in cost per capita for personal health care for the elderly from just prior to Medicare to several years after Medicare, as seen in Table 4.9, we see a pattern of increase of approximately $100 per capita per year, from $445 in fiscal 1966 to $1,218 in fiscal 1974. Hospital and nursing home care showed the steepest rates of increase, from $177.84 and $68.39 in 1966 to $573.18 and $289.10, respectively, in 1974 (Brehm, 1978).

These data on changes in the rates of utilization suggest that the explicit intent of Medicare, that is, to reduce the financial barrier to obtaining medical services, was achieved only in part. A greater number of elderly persons are obtaining needed services. The trends, however, belie the initial fear that health resources would be "swamped" by excessive demand (Munan, Vobecky, and Kelly, 1974). Of increasing concern is the cost of even maintaining services at this level when all indications are that demand will increase along with growth in the size of the elderly population. This concern is not limited to absolute costs but also relative costs in relation to total national expenditures for personal health care. Prior to 1967, the percentage of total personal health care expenditures paid by Federal dollars was 25 percent at its highest. After Medicare was initiated, expenditures from this program alone, as a percentage of the total for personal health care, rose from 31.6 percent in 1967 to 42.0 percent in 1975. Consideration of this trend in light of policy on resource allocation raises ethical questions (Jonsen, 1976).

The data on use and cost of health services indicate that the increases in demand and expenditures for such services over the first ten years of Medicare were primarily the result of changes in patterns of use of these services and of dramatic increases in their cost. The history of increases in the levels of use and the percentages of the gross national product as well as per capita expenditures devoted to health care attest to the influence of Medicare on these increases.

AVAILABILITY

Our assessment of the impact of Medicare on the availability of health services for the elderly will focus on the development and use of alternate levels of care. Specifically, we are concerned with skilled nursing facilities (extended care facilities) and home health services, use of which can be paid for by the program. The stimulation of these care modalities and their use was intended under the program as a means to reduce use of more expensive forms of care.

As an additional issue, we will also review the change in nursing home use from before to after Medicare. While general nursing home use is not reimbursable under the program, these institutions do primarily serve the

TABLE 4.9: Estimated per Capita Personal Health Care Expenditures for Population 65 and over, 1966–74

Year	Hospital Care	Physicians' Services	Nursing Home Care	Total
1966	$177.84	$89.57	$68.39	$445.25
1970	375.13	141.60	162.76	828.31
1974	573.18	182.14	289.10	1,217.84

Source: U.S. Department of Health, Education, and Welfare, 1976a.

elderly population. Medicaid payments are available for nursing home care if the aged individual qualifies under this means-tested program. Medicare benefits are available only if the institution has a unit that is certified as a skilled nursing facility and if the elderly patient qualifies for reimbursement for a stay in such a facility. The reimbursement, of course, is limited to the relatively short period of stay covered under the program.

If the data reported above are a reasonable indication of the pattern of increased use of hospital in-patient facilities, then the use of extended care facilities and home health services, as the alternatives to the use of hospital services, should also have increased if these less expensive care modalities were being used appropriately.

However, Medicare program data show that the number of admissions to skilled nursing facilities peaked in 1969, one year after this part of the program was initiated, and has declined since. In 1968, there were 22.7 admissions to SNFs per 1,000 enrollees. This rose to 26.3 per 1,000 in 1969 and was reported as 19.5 per 1,000 in 1974. SNF admissions as a percentage of hospital admissions rose to 8.6 percent in 1969; in 1974 the comparable figure was 6.1 percent. Other data reveal that "denial of SNF benefits was considerable during Medicare's first decade and that approval of post-hospital SNF care has gone primarily to cases with long hospital stays" (Gornick, 1976, p. 11).

As can be seen in Table 4.10, skilled nursing facilities have consistently been used more by women than by men, and the levels of reimbursement per person served and enrolled have been higher for women. However, between 1967 and 1976 there was a decrease, for both sexes, of 32 percent in the number of persons served per 1,000 enrollees, and of 12 percent in the reimbursement per person enrolled.

Home health services, like skilled nursing facilities, have also been used more by women, and women have had higher levels of reimbursement for these services. However, use of these services increased more for men than for women from 1967 to 1976, so that the gap between them on this measure narrowed considerably (Table 4.11). Use of these two services, skilled nursing facilities and home health services, accounts for the smallest

TABLE 4.10: Use of Skilled Nursing Facilities (Extended Care Facilities) under HI for Persons 65 and over, 1967 and 1976

Usage Indicator	1967	1976	Percent Change, 1967–76
Persons served per 1,000 enrolled			
Total	18.2	12.5	−31.3
Male	15.2	10.4	−31.6
Female	20.3	13.9	−31.5
Reimbursement total (in $1,000)			
Total	$274,295	$283,390	+ 3.3
Male	91,801	90,552	− 1.4
Female	182,494	192,839	+ 5.7
Reimbursement per person served			
Total	$774.41	$990.80	+27.9
Male	732.30	934.30	+27.6
Female	797.48	1,019.77	+27.9
Reimbursement per person enrolled			
Total	$14.07	$12.36	−12.2
Male	11.14	9.71	−12.8
Female	16.22	14.18	−12.6

Source: U.S. Department of Health, Education, and Welfare, *Medicare 1967* and *Medicare 1975–76.*

program pieces, in that, as of 1976, these services were used by the smallest number of persons per 1,000 enrolled and had the lowest levels of reimbursement. Nonetheless, home health services, unlike skilled nursing facilities, showed an increased use over the decade, more under HI than under SMI.

The data collected for the Kansas City area indicate the total number of ECF beds in both hospital and nursing home-based ECFs declined from 1,045 to 749 between 1968–69 and 1970–71. This was a drop from 8.8 to 6.4 beds per 1,000 persons aged 65 or over. While the number of beds per 1,000 persons 65 and over was less in Kansas City than in the United States as a whole, the pattern of decrease in total beds and in beds per 1,000 aged people was the same in both cases.

Although fewer ECF than nursing home beds were available in Kansas City, neither setting had an average occupancy rate in 1971 that reached 50 percent. Thus, there seems to have been a sizable excess of ECF-certified

TABLE 4.11: Use of Home Health Services under HI and SMI for Persons 65 and over, 1967 and 1976

Usage Indicator	Home Health Services under HI			Home Health Services under SMI		
	1967	*1976*	*Percent change, 1967-76*	*1967*	*1976*	*Percent change, 1967-76*
Persons served per 1,000 enrolled						
Total	6.5	17.8	+173.9	6.6	8.6	+30.3
Male	5.4	16.2	+200.0	4.4	6.8	+54.6
Female	7.3	18.9	+158.9	8.2	9.8	+19.5
Reimbursement total (in $1,000)						
Total	$25,783	$193,184	+649.3	$17,061	$74,667	+337.7
Male	8,569	71,484	+734.2	4,613	23,224	+403.4
Female	17,215	121,700	+606.9	12,447	51,443	+313.3
Reimbursement per person served						
Total	$204.45	$473.89	+131.8	$144.80	387.00	+167.3
Male	192.75	473.47	+145.6	139.07	379.85	+173.1
Female	210.82	474.13	+124.9	147.04	390.31	+165.4
Reimbursement per person enrolled						
Total	$1.32	$8.43	+538.6	$0.95	$3.33	+250.5
Male	1.04	7.67	+637.5	0.61	2.57	+321.3
Female	1.53	8.95	+485.0	1.20	3.84	+220.0

Source: U.S. Department of Health, Education, and Welfare, *Medicare 1967* and *Medicare 1975–76.*

beds that were not being used, despite the decline in the number of such beds. This decline is especially significant because extended care is a concept and practice directly associated with Medicare. All expectations would have been for continued growth of this level of care, as had been evident in the first days of the program (Coe, Brehm, and Peterson, 1974).

As with ECFs, payment for home health services was provided as part of the effort to promote the availability and use of appropriate alternative care levels for older people. Some home care programs were already in existence, such as visiting nurse associations and public health nursing from health departments. Medicare provided the stimulus for development or expansion of such services. The trend in Kansas City followed this pattern in that there was a consistent increase from 1966 through 1971 in the total number of visits made by home health agencies. However, as Table 4.12 shows, the number of visits to persons 65 and over, the rate of visits per 1,000 population in this age group, and the percentage of all visits that were covered by Medicare peaked between 1968 and 1970 and declined abruptly in 1971 (Coe et al., 1974). The overall data from the Medicare program confirm this pattern, in that the percentage of program reimbursement for home health care under both HI and SMI peaked in 1969 and then dropped through 1972. In both cases, however, use has been rapidly accelerated since (Gornick, 1976).

For Kansas City, the data through 1971 show a consistent upward trend in the rate of home health visits per 1,000 of total population. The implication is not that these agencies reduced their services in 1971, but that for a period of time they were less directed toward Medicare beneficiaries. The overall program data indicate this pattern changed for home health care use, unlike SNFs, but do not suggest there was a concurrent drop in hospital in-patient care. The pattern of reduction in average length of stay has been fairly consistent.

There were changes in the Medicare reimbursement policy in the period under review. While there was no change in the legislative definition for use of SNFs or home health services, there was a more stringent administrative interpretation of justifications. As a result, approvals for payment were more difficult to obtain. This had a negative effect on the finances of the providers because it resulted in disapprovals after services were provided. This administrative tightening-up was based on concern for the level of total expenditures under Medicare and for the appropriateness of the use of these alternatives to continued in-patient care. If SNFs had been being used as originally planned, their use would have significantly reduced the length of hospital stays. Under these circumstances, less expensive treatment levels would have been used and it is doubtful that a cutback in SNF use would have been seen as a way to save Medicare funds. Pressure might then have been applied for increased, not decreased, use of lower levels of care when appropriate, to save program funds that were spent on in-patient hospital

TABLE 4.12: Use of Home Health Agencies in Kansas City, 1966–71

Usage Indicator	1966	1967	1968	1969	1970	1971
Total visits	40,556	50,417	65,982	66,228	75,279	78,787
Visits paid for through Medicare	3,240	25,482	38,632	39,326	39,566	35,773
Percent Medicare visits	8%	51%	59%	59%	54%	45%
Rate of total visits per 1,000 of total population	34	41	53	53	60	62
Rate of Medicare visits per 1,000 of population 65 or over	29	227	340	341	338	301

Source: Coe, et al., 1973, Table III-2 and Figure 1, App. B.

85

care. The probability is that the administrative pressure to keep acute-care beds filled resulted in a lack of appropriate use of these facilities that were to reduce the length of hospital stays. In other words, "the medical care delivery system might not have been making appropriate use of alternative and less expensive levels of care to reduce use of hospital facilities but might have been using these services in considerable measure for patients who would have been discharged from the hospital at the same point in time in any event" (Coe et al., 1974, p. 254).

Nursing and Personal Care Homes

Nursing and personal care homes are a special category of health-related facility used primarily by the aged. In 1963, there were slightly over 500,000 residents in nursing and personal care homes in this country. Of these, 12 percent were under age 65, and 70% were 75 and over. There were 8 residents per 1,000 population for those 65–74, and 57 per 1,000 for those 75 and over. By 1969, a few years after the Medicare and Medicaid programs started, the age distribution of residents in these homes had showed only minor change since 1963. However, the number of residents per 1,000 population was dramatically higher, particularly among the very old. It had increased from 57 to 77 per 1,000 population for those 75 and over. For those 65–74, the rate had gone up from 8 to 11 per 1,000 population (Brehm, 1978).

In 1963, 68 percent of nursing home residents 65 and over were women. In 1974, 72 percent were women, compared with approximately 59 percent of the general population 65 and over in that year. The average number of residents per 1,000 population was higher for women than for men in groups aged 65 and over and 75 and over in 1963 and 1969, and increased for both sexes between 1963 and 1969. For those 75 and over, the rate was 40 per 1,000 population for men and 69 per 1,000 population for women in 1963. These rates increased to 52 per 1,000 population for men and 92 per 1,000 population for women in 1969 (NCHS, 1965 and 1973).

In absolute numbers, the population of these homes had grown by over 300,000 persons between 1963 and 1969, to a total of over 800,000 residents. The vast majority of this increase was based on a change in pattern of use and much less on an increase in the size of the aged population. By 1974, there were over 1,000,000 residents in nursing and personal care homes (NCHS, 1977). Again, the increase is not based on population increase.

The data for Kansas City indicate an increase in the number of nursing home beds over the period of study. However, this increase in beds was accompanied by a small decrease in the number of homes, indicating a move toward larger homes, some of which were part of a nationwide chain. The bed to aged population ratio more than kept pace with population growth, rising from 41 per 1,000 older people in 1967 to 48 per 1,000 in 1971. Over half of these homes were licensed as practical nursing homes in 1971; slightly less than 40 percent were licensed as professional, skilled homes. The occupancy rate for non-ECF nursing home beds, unlike ECF beds, remained between 85 percent and 89 percent from 1967 through 1971. Apparently, there was no decrease in the traditional use of nursing homes (Coe et al., 1974).

COORDINATION OF HEALTH SERVICES FOR THE AGED

In attempting to assess the presumed impact of Medicare on the system for delivery of health services, we will focus our attention on the data collected in the Kansas City studies for the three time periods starting just before the program began and ending in 1971. This allows us to view the effect of Medicare on the workings of the system at the local level, where health services for the aged are actually delivered. At the time of the study, Kansas City's demographic, social, and economic characteristics were not particularly different from national patterns.

Analysis of the data for the period between 1966 and 1968 indicated:

(1) There was virtually no planned coordination of health care facilities in any of the communities studied; (2) Medicare was used as a justification for expanding short-term acute-care capacities of hospitals; (3) the program had little effect on the way in which doctors practice medicine, but broadened the doctor's role in the health care scheme; and (4) Medicare had legitimated and encouraged some expansion of a needed service—home health care (Coe et al., 1974, p. 232).

Very little change was seen in these first two years in the provision of services to older people or the utilization of services by them. The follow-up in 1971 was to determine if the expectation that Medicare would stimulate changes in the provision and organization of services and in referral patterns had been realized.

The expectation was for an expansion in the range and amount of services. In addition to SNFs, home health agencies, and nursing homes, as discussed earlier, changes were looked for in physicians' office practices and hospitals. Additionally, it was anticipated that an expansion of services to make them more comprehensive would require organizational changes to link providers more closely through voluntary coordination and cooperation. Referral patterns directed at providing alternative levels of care were expected to develop (Coe et al., 1974).

Health Services in the Community

The entry point for an elderly individual into treatment by a community's health system is the practicing physician. In 1970, there were 1.28 physicians for every 1,000 people in Kansas City, about the national average. This represented a slight drop in the physician/population ratio from 1.30 per 1,000 in 1965. If osteopaths are included, the decline was even more significant: from 1.51 physicians per 1,000 population in 1965 to 1.44 in 1970. The proportion of general practitioners dropped from 18.4 percent to 13.2 percent in that time. The decrease was accounted for by an increase in the proportion of medical specialists, with little change in the proportion of surgical specialists.

The Kansas City physicians interviewed in 1971 reported a slightly lower level of office visits compared with the physicians sampled in 1968. However, they also reported an increase in the percentage of their patients who were elderly and an increase in office visits by this group since the beginning of Medicare. These data correspond only in part with data from a sample of older people, to be reviewed in greater detail in the next chapter. The older people reported a decline in physician office visits from 1966 to 1968 and an increase in 1971, but to less than the 1966 level.

In response to a series of questions about alternatives to prolonged hospital care, most of the physicians interviewed in 1971 said they considered an ECF or home health services an acceptable alternative to prolonged hospitalization. As can be seen in Table 4.13, the primary reasons given were related to lower cost, more appropriate care level, and the freeing of acute-care hospital beds.

Of the physicians interviewed, 60 percent claimed they used ECFs as an alternative to prolonged hospital care for their older patients; 56 percent claimed they used home health care for this purpose. However, as can be seen in Table 4.14, few of these physicians reported they treated patients anywhere other than their private offices or in the hospital. Over 60 percent of the physicians said "none" to separate questions on the number of house calls, nursing home calls, or ECF calls last week (Coe et al., 1974).

Most physicians (69 percent) said Medicare had made changes in the availability of health services in the community, but primarily in terms of financial availability. The overwhelming majority (82 percent) also said Medicare had made changes in the use of services, particularly an increased use of hospitals and physicians.

In response to a question on the best way to increase physician services, few of the physicians mentioned any changes in the structure or delivery of health services, including increasing the number or use of paramedics (see Table 4.15). "In other words, while physicians are aware of the alternatives and express some agreement with the possibilities for co-ordination of services, they have not significantly altered their methods of treating patients because of the Medicare program" (Coe et al., 1974, p. 244).

Between 1966 and 1971, there was an increase from 5.3 to 5.7 hospital beds per 1,000 population in Kansas City. The percent of all admissions for

TABLE 4.13: Attitudes toward Use of ECF and Home Health Services among Kansas City Physicians, 1971 (in percent)

Response	Is ECF an Acceptable Alternative to Hospital?	Is HHS an Acceptable Alternative to Hospital Care?	Is HHS an Acceptable Alternative to ECF Care?
Yes	74.5	69 1	50.9
No	18.2	21.8	36.4
NA	7.2	9.1	12.7
Total (N = 55)	100.0	100.0	100.0
	Why (Why Not)?	*Why (Why Not)?*	*Why (Why Not)?*
	Less expensive; reduce cost — 30.9	Low-level care needed — 30.9	Where lower-level care sufficient — 21.8
	More appropriate care level — 20.0	Recovery at home faster — 20.0	Home care not good enough — 16.4

TABLE 4.13 (continued)

Why (Why Not)?		Why (Why Not)?		Why (Why Not)?	
Free acute hospital beds	10.9	Less expensive; lower cost	10.9	Home setting good for treatment	10.9
ECFs over-utilized	10.9	Free hospital for acute care	10.9	Home care not necessary	5.5
Not enough flexibility	9.1	Unnecessary if well enough to be home	5.5	If patient's condition warrants it	3.6
Economically unsound	1.8	Other	16.4	NA	41.8
Other	7.3	NA	18.1		
NA	9.1				
Total	100.0	Total	100.0	Total	100.0

NA = not answered.
Source: Coe, Brehm, and Peterson, 1974, Table 6. Used by permission.

TABLE 4.14: **Number of House Calls, Nursing Home Calls, ECF Calls, and Visits to Other Places Last Week by Kansas City Physicians, 1971**

	House Calls	Nursing Home Calls	ECF Calls	Visits to Other Places
None	63.6	61.8	65.5	49.1
1–5	12.7	12.7	5.5	—
6 or more	1.8	3.6	1.8	3.6
NA	21.8	21.8	27.3	47.3
Total (N = 55)	100.0	100.0	100.0	100.0

— = no response in category.

NA = not answered.

Note: Figures indicate percent of physicians having made that type of call in the last week.

Source: Coe et al., 1974, Table 8. Used by permission.

patients age 65 and over rose from 22.4 percent before Medicare to 27.6 percent in 1967 and 30.2 percent in 1968. It dropped to 26.1 percent in 1970. However, data from the survey of the elderly in Kansas City show a higher percentage hospitalized during 1970 than during 1968.

Interagency Coordination

Cooperation among the health facilities in Kansas City did not increase significantly from 1968 to 1971. However, there was a reasonable level of

TABLE 4.15: **Kansas City Physician Opinions on the Best Way to Increase Physician Services, 1971**

Possible Actions	Percent Agreeing
Increase number of M.D.s	32.7
Reduce paper-work; use credit cards	10.9
Keep service at present level; no increase necessary	9.1
Change geographic distribution of M.D. services	7.3
Promote group practice	5.5
Police utilization; screen out well patients; reduce overutilization	5.5
Expand insurance coverage	3.6
Increase number and use of paramedics	1.8
No answer/doesn't apply	23.6
Total (N=55)	100.0

Source: Coe, et al., 1974, Table 11. Used by permission.

cooperation. About 6 out of 10 hospitals had formal transfer agreements with nursing home ECFs in both 1968 and 1971. There were 5 home health service agencies in operation, and few hospitals had any plans to develop their own home health services. However, the proportion of the 32 Kansas City area hospitals with a home health services coordinator on the staff dropped by almost half, from 56 percent to 33 percent, between 1968 and 1971.

An official comprehensive health planning (CHP) agency was established in the Kansas City area between the 1968 and 1971 rounds of data collection. The 1971 survey asked about this agency. It is possible to draw some conclusions about increased coordination of health services from these data. Table 4.16 shows that more hospital managers than other health personnel surveyed were aware of the agency's existence and thought it was doing an effective job. These results are not surprising, given that this agency, like most of its counterparts, devoted most of its time to matters involving provision of hospital services. Operators of privately owned nursing homes would have little direct reason to know about or be influenced by a CHP agency. Home health agency directors also would not seem directly involved with hospital-oriented planning groups. However, barely half of the study doctors knew about the agency. This seems unusual since they represent the first step of formal care. Furthermore, those who

TABLE 4.16: **Knowledge and Evaluation of Comprehensive Health Planning Agency, Kansas City (in percent)**

Response	Physicians	Hospital Administrators	Nursing Home Operators	Home Health Directors
Is there a CHP Agency here?				
Yes	56	97	24	100
No	7	3	20	—
Don't know	37	—	56	—
Total	100 (N=55)	100 (N=32)	100 (N=80)	100 (N=5)
Is CHP effective?				
Yes	24	44	11	—
No	22	32	7	—
Don't know	54	24	82	100
Total	100 (N=55)	100 (N=32)	100 (N=80)	100 (N=5)

— = No responses in category.
Source: Coe, et al., 1973, Table II-2.

knew about the agency were almost equally divided in their opinion of it. None of this suggests strong backing for an agency designed to bring about a new organization of health resources (Coe et al., 1974).

When we review perceptions of the present status of health resources in Kansas City, as shown in Table 4.17, two things are apparent: all respondents except home health agency directors tended to view resources for the younger population as more adequate than those for the elderly. More importantly, the proportion of physicians who viewed the then current resources as adequate was much higher than for any other kind of provider. In addition, much of the fact that resources were perceived as available was associated with Medicare; 69 percent of the physicians, 60 percent of the nursing home managers, and 47 percent of the hospital administrators tied the Medicare program to changes in availability of health services.

Despite this generally high level of satisfaction with the adequacy of community resources, there was a perception of need for more long-term care facilities and services among all respondents. In the 1968 survey of facility managers, 60 percent of the hospital administrators said they had plans to build or expand their facilities, and 64 percent planned to expand

**TABLE 4.17: Perception of Adequacy of Community Health
Resources in Kansas City, Missouri**

Are resources adequate?	For Residents Age 65 and Over (in percent)			
	Physicians	Hospital Administrators	Nursing Home Operators	Home Health Directors
Yes	64	31	28	—
No	25	56	54	100
Don't know	11	12	18	—
Total	100	100	100	100
N	55	32	80	5

Are resources adequate?	For Residents Under Age 65 (in percent)			
	Physicians	Hospital Administrators	Nursing Home Operators	Home Health Directors
Yes	71	31	33	—
No	13	50	33	100
Don't know	16	19	34	—
Total	100	100	100	100
N	55	32	80	5

Source: Coe, et al., 1973, Table II-1.

their services. These planned increases were mostly for acute medical service (36 percent). Rehabilitation and long-term care were far down the list (12 percent). However, by 1971 only one hospital had expanded its physical plant and eight others (25 percent) had increased their services. All but two of these were for long-term care or rehabilitation services.

The most obvious changes for hospitals and nursing homes were in staff size. Half of the hospitals in Kansas City added staff between 1968 and 1971. For 13 hospitals the increase was in the administrative staff, primarily to process Medicare-related matters. For three, staff increases were mostly for direct patient services, that is, nursing, dietetics, and pharmacy.

The provision of health care services in Kansas City did not change much between 1968 and 1971 despite the fact that most area providers *perceived* Medicare as having had a strong effect on development of new services. Most of the earlier stated plans for physical plant expansion had not been implemented. Only a small proportion of institutions increased their services. However, most *service program* expansion was in the area of rehabilitation and chronic care, rather than acute medical and surgical services as was the case between 1966 and 1968. There was a reduction in capacity to provide extended care services. In sum, the Medicare program clearly influenced the provision of health services in Kansas City, but not to the degree perceived by practitioners or expected in terms of anticipated changes (Coe et al., 1974).

Preliminary Conclusions

It had been expected that community health resource managers would respond initially to the anticipated increased demand for specialized health care services for the elderly by reallocating their present resources. Additionally, it was expected that the need for collaboration among the various providers to effect more comprehensive services would lead to greater coordination and better distribution of health services. Local physician groups were expected to play a leading role in assessing the need for such collaboration and in effecting the means for achieving it. This general prediction concerning the impact of Medicare on health care delivery systems in local communities served as a focus for analysis in this part of the investigation.

The assessment that covered the period from 1966 to 1968 showed that some hospitals, home health care agencies, nursing homes, and other facilities had shifted their resources or added to their capacity in response to Medicare. However, such changes were according to decisions made on the part of individual organizations, with little reference to a community health care system. Medicare, along with other inducements, led to an expansion of the traditional acute-care capacities of hospitals. There was some development of extended care facilities. However, physicians saw little effect from

Medicare on their practices and saw little need for reorganization of community health resources; some were beginning to utilize ECFs or home health care for their patients.

One important difference in the findings from the 1971 follow-up compared with the 1968 study was the general lack of additional change or plans for growth. In the initial period of Medicare services many institutions were planning expansion of the physical plant and increases in staff. By 1971, it was clear that few earlier plans had been implemented, and that little further expansion of facilities or increases in staff and services related to Medicare or the needs of older patients was planned.

Between 1968 and 1971, there was continued development of larger and better-equipped nursing homes, and an increase in the total number of beds. Significantly, from the standpoint of continuity of care for older persons and the intent of the Medicare legislation to encourage alternative lower-cost care modes, the number of extended care facilities and their utilization declined during the 1968–1971 period. In effect, the initial beginning of a system to facilitate continuity of care simply had not developed in any measure proportionate to the need.

Physicians revealed little change in style or organization of practice. The overwhelming majority agreed with the concepts of extended care and home health services as suitable alternatives to prolonged hospitalization when appropriate for the case. However, few used these resources even though the full range of services was available to them. "The private office and the acute hospital continue to be the dominant settings for care of the elderly, while alternative forms or settings for care remain largely outside the sphere of the organization of the community's resources" (Coe et al., 1974, p. 262). Physicians have not acted to facilitate the coordination of health care services in the community even though they remain the key to the delivery of these services. The findings from the Kansas City analysis can be briefly summarized as follows: "Medicare has not (nor has anything else) appreciably altered the organization of health services in the study community" (Coe et al., 1974, p. 262).

The unavoidable conclusion is that the implicit intent of the legislation was not realized. The assessment of the interrelationships among providers indicated no real movement toward a comprehensive system of care for the aged. If anything, it was business as usual, with an improved guarantee of payment.

5

HOW THE ELDERLY
PERCEIVE AND RESPOND
TO MEDICARE

In the last chapter we assessed two aspects of the impact of Medicare. First, we reviewed the changes in use and cost of health care for the aged from before to after the program started. Second, the program's impact on the health services system in terms of organization and delivery of care in one geographic area was analyzed. In this chapter we want to assess the reactions of the aged to Medicare in the same geographic area, as the target population.

Medicare did have some impact, if only temporary, on the development and organization of a community's health services. As we illustrated in the preceding chapter, the explicit intent of the legislation to reduce the financial barriers to obtaining care was evidenced by increased utilization of certain services by the elderly, but the greatest impact was in the huge increases in the costs of care and of operating the program. The implicit intent of the program, namely, to create new services, was also partly fulfilled especially in intermediate or extended care and in the growth of home health agencies, but the relationship of the program to these services after the initial stimulus was not sustained. Increased coordination and collaborative organization of health services in the community, as an implicit goal, were not achieved, for the reasons noted earlier. The perspective of the providers varied depending upon their role in the health system. Physicians, the key to any coordinated process, saw little need to alter their customary practice organization to care for the elderly. Hospital administrators responded initially with plans for changes in programs and facilities, but soon became more occupied with costs of care and reimbursement mechanisms. Directors of extended care facilities, nursing homes, and home health agencies also held views and dealt with problems related almost entirely to their position in the health organizational structure of the community and not to the system as a whole.

The impact of Medicare on community health services can be viewed from the perspective of the consumer, the elderly in the community, in two ways: first, in terms of the impact on the elderly themselves, that is, changes in their health perceptions and behaviors; and second, in terms of evaluation by the elderly of the effects of Medicare on the health services delivery system in the community. In the first case, Medicare as an innovation in payment for medical care was expected to produce a change in the definition of health status. Over time, conditions associated with aging would be expected to become defined as illness rather than "normal" aging. Thus, a chronic illness would provide a legitimate reason for seeking care. As this took place *and* financial barriers were lowered, the utilization of care services should increase. Increased care should be associated with an improvement in perception of well-being, representing a distinct change from the pre-Medicare pattern of association of high utilization with low perceived health status.

The second type of evaluation, the elderly's perception of the adequacy of community health resources to deal with their problems, is more difficult to assess, but also relates directly to perception of changes in the organization of community health services resulting from the Medicare program. The explicit intent of the legislation to increase the affordability of care can be measured in the perceptions of the elderly consumer. Similarly, the implicit objectives of increasing availability and accessibility through reorganization, and creation of new roles and new services can be also assessed by responses from the elderly consumer. These perceptions were explored through interviews with elderly residents in Kansas City, the largest of our study sites, using separate samples at times, as described in Chapter 1.

ATTITUDES TOWARD THE MEDICARE PROGRAM

One of the major changes was the increase in the early years of the program in favorable attitudes toward Medicare. In response to the question, "Do you think Medicare is a good idea?" the percentage of Kansas City respondents who said "yes" increased from 73 percent in 1966, to 88 percent in 1968. In the last (1971) survey, 87 percent responded affirmatively to the same question, 3 percent said "no," and 10 percent were "not sure." There had been no change since the previous data collection period. As is apparent from Table 5.1, the total sample is reflected by the categories of each of the independent variables.

Although general approval of Medicare did not increase from 1968 to 1971, the reasons for approval have altered somewhat. The most frequently cited reason for approval of the program in 1971 was that it "provides care for those who need it" (40 percent). In 1968 the most common reason was that it "provides money for those who need it," which was mentioned second most often in 1971 (35 percent). The financial benefit was mentioned by 17 percent *fewer* respondents in 1971, while focus on the hospital and on the

TABLE 5.1: **Percentage of Respondents Who Answered "Yes" to "Do You Think Medicare is a Good Idea?" by Selected Dimensions**

Dimension	1966	1968	1971
All dimensions	73	88	87
Occupation			
White-collar	74	87	89
Blue-collar	75	87	86
Perceived health status			
Very good	75	89	90
Good	73	90	84
Fair	74	86	91
Poor	70	84	81
Preventive-care orientation			
Checkups	71	89	91
Only when sick	73	88	85
Never go	66	76	78
Perceived Adequacy of Income			
Comfortable	75	89	87
Adequate	71	89	87
Inadequate	72	82	85
Age			
60–64	70	86	81
65–69	75	90	89
70–74	75	89	92
75 or over	72	87	87
Sex			
Male	79	89	87
Female	71	87	87

Source: Coe, et al., 1973, Table IV-3.

program in general increased the most. Hospital care was mentioned by 22 percent; 18 percent considered Medicare "a good idea." The shift in emphasis from "providing money" to "providing care" may reflect an increased familiarity by the older population with the actual operations of the Medicare program.

The small number of respondents who could give a reason when they did not believe Medicare was a good idea most often (29 percent) cited "inefficient operation," which was not even mentioned in previous surveys. On the other hand, major reasons given before, that is, overutilization and poor insurance program, were not mentioned in 1971. However, the 10 percent who were "unsure" whether Medicare was a good idea gave their reasons as lack of knowledge (49 percent), high cost (19 percent), and poor coverage (10 percent).

To the direct question "Has Medicare changed your feelings about your sense of security?" 54 percent of the 1971 sample replied "yes," compared with 50 percent in 1968; the question was not asked in 1966. Of the 380 respondents who replied this way, the great majority (96 percent) indicated it had increased their feelings of security. Among the reasons given were (1) access to doctors, hospitals, and so on (45 percent); (2) provision of money for care (39 percent); and (3) psychological factors, such as relief from worry (34 percent). In 1968, when the same coding categories were used, more respondents cited provision of money (54 percent) than access to services (39 percent).

It can be concluded that the overwhelming majority of respondents approved strongly of the Medicare program. Medicare had increased the feeling of security in the older population and their feeling that they had access to medical services. Some concern about "inefficiency" in the Medicare program had emerged, while concerns about overutilization had declined.

ATTITUDES TOWARD HEALTH CARE
PROVIDERS AND RESOURCES

Another major line of inquiry involved changes in attitudes of older people toward hospitals, nursing homes, and physicians. The measurement of attitudes was accomplished by means of a battery of statements with which the respondent was asked if she or he agreed or disagreed. Ten of these statements assess the degree of faith in physicians, essentially a measure of trust in science-based medical care. Two other sets, each with four comparable questions, were designed to tap attitudes towards hospitals, with which about 18 percent had had some experience in 1971, and nursing homes, with which almost no one in the sample had had any experience.

Attitude toward Hospitals and Nursing Homes

Data on attitudes toward hospitals are shown in Table 5.2. Most respondents felt that hospitals give good care and that, for serious illnesses, hospital care is better than treatment at home. Even for these items, however, the proportion of favorable responses declined in the last time period, while the percentage of unfavorable responses increased.

By far the most dramatic change can be seen in the final item relating to cost of care, specifically to a perception that the care received in hospitals is worth the cost, that is, the actual charges to the patient. In the first place, more respondents held an opinion about costs by 1971. Secondly, this was

TABLE 5.2: **Attitudes toward Hospitals, Kansas City (in percent)**

Attitudinal Statement	1966		1968		1971	
	Agree	*Disagree*	*Agree*	*Disagree*	*Agree*	*Disagree*
Most hospitals give good care to patients. (Agree)*	87	6	91	5	88	9
If a person needs a lot of medical care, he/she is better off in a hospital than at home. (Agree)	73	18	79	18	74	24
In the hospital, younger patients get more attention and care than older ones. (Disagree)	14	60	16	64	18	69
In general, hospital charges are fair for the services a patient gets. (Agree)	47	34	38	48	30	63

*Favorable response in parentheses.
Source: Coe, et al., 1973, Table IV-4.

the only item for which by 1968 there had been an increase in unfavorable response over 1966. Third, and most important, by 1971 unfavorable responses were given twice as frequently as favorable replies. These findings suggest that respondents were increasingly focusing on costs as a source of discontent with the delivery of medical care in general and the Medicare program in particular.

Items somewhat comparable in content were used to measure attitudes toward nursing homes. Although in all three samples attitudes toward nursing homes were more negative than toward hospitals, the direction of change was similar. Most respondents felt that nursing homes were preferable to imposing on a relative if one is unable to care for oneself, but the percentage holding this view declined from 1968 to 1971. No other item for nursing homes received a favorable response from a majority of respondents.

As is indicated in Table 5.3, a larger proportion disagreed than agreed that nursing homes give good care. The negative perspective on nursing homes in general is expressed even more forcefully with regard to recovering from an operation. A person's own home was chosen twice as often as a nursing home. Finally, again, respondents reacted sharply to costs of care in nursing homes, the majority disagreeing that charges were fair for the care received. This was a significant increase over 1968.

Scores on individual items were combined to form indexes of attitudes toward hospitals and nursing homes. These data are found in Table 5.4. Clearly there was an overall decline in scores for both types of institutions, although much of the loss from the most favorable response for hospitals may be derived from attitudes that were only slightly less favorable. However, there were slight increases also in the least favorable responses toward hospitals.

For nursing homes, the trend in attitudes is clearly negative and of much greater magnitude than for hospitals. Taken together, these data on attitudes, combined with statements about the Medicare program noted earlier, seem to suggest there was growing concern from the older population about the health care system.

Faith in Physicians

Responses to the items in the index of faith in physicians are shown in Table 5.5. Initial inspection of trends for these items would seem to yield mixed results. That is, for some items, like the first one shown, "Patients should follow the doctor's orders even if they are not sure he is right," there was a decline by 1971 in favorable response, a reversal of the earlier trend. In 1971, fewer respondents agreed with the statement (a favorable response) and a larger proportion disagreed than in 1968, although the change from

TABLE 5.3: Attitudes toward Nursing Homes, Kansas City (in percent)

Attitudinal Statement	1966		1968		1971	
	Agree	*Disagree*	*Agree*	*Disagree*	*Agree*	*Disagree*
A person who can no longer care for himself is better off in a nursing home than in the home of a relative. (Agree)*	62	22	71	19	67	26
People can get good care in a nursing home. (Agree)	33	25	45	25	35	42
After an operation, an older patient can recover more quickly in a nursing home than in his own home. (Agree)	20	52	24	55	22	65
In general, nursing home costs are fair for the services a patient gets. (Agree)	25	23	28	32	20	51

*Favorable response in parentheses.
Source: Coe, et al., 1973, table IV-5.

TABLE 5.4: Index of Attitudes toward Hospitals and Nursing Homes (in percent)

Index Scores	Hospitals			Nursing Homes		
	1966	1968	1971	1966	1968	1971
1.80–1.99 (Favorable)	47	36	24	31	27	13
1.60–1.79	32	41	45	17	24	20
1.40–1.59	13	15	22	19	17	21
1.20–1.39	5	6	7	12	18	22
1.00–1.19 (Unfavorable)	3	2	3	22	16	24
Total	100	100	100	100	100	100
N	861	704	699	816	689	688
Mean score	1.73	1.71	1.66	1.55	1.56	1.45

Source: Coe, et al., 1973, table IV-6.

103

TABLE 5.5: Attitudes toward Physicians, Kansas City, 1966, 1968, and 1971 (in percent)

Attitudinal Statement	1966		1968		1971	
	Agree	Disagree	Agree	Disagree	Agree	Disagree
Patients should follow the doctor's orders even if they are not sure he is right. (Agree)*	81	12	88	9	84	15
Doctors usually give better care to younger patients than to older ones. (Disagree)	14	68	16	70	16	76
Even if a patient can't pay, a doctor will give good treatment. (Agree)	63	12	67	15	64	21
Doctors don't give as much time to older patients as they do younger ones. (Disagree)	17	62	17	67	18	73
If a doctor can't help you, he'll tell you that right away. (Agree)	58	23	61	27	56	36

Whether you pay them or not, doctors will give you as much time and attention as you need. (Agree)	49	23	55	25	53	32
For some kinds of sickness, a doctor is not always the best person to go to for help. (Disagree)	25	56	25	64	25	65
People should try out different doctors to see which ones they will like the best. (Disagree)	45	45	45	50	46	51
A person usually knows his/her own health status better than most doctors do. (Disagree)	48	42	54	41	56	42
Most doctors are interested only in the patient's illness and not in the patient's other problems. (Disagree)	54	29	64	24	66	28

*Favorable response is in parentheses.
Source: Coe, et al. 1973, table IV-7.

1966 to 1968 had been in the other direction. Similar results are seen with three other items (numbers 3, 5, and 6). Important but less dramatic shifts can also be found for statements like "A person usually knows his own health condition better than most doctors do," and "Most doctors are interested only in the patients' illness and not in other problems." In these two items (and number 8), there was a slight increase in unfavorable response, but little or no change in favorable response, from 1968 to 1971 and, in some cases, since 1966. For the remaining three items (numbers 2, 4, and 7), the trend after 1966 was toward an increase in favorable response with little or no change in unfavorable response. It is interesting to note that two of the latter statements explicitly refer to perception of differential treatment because of age. Clearly the older respondents did not believe they received poorer care because they are older.

In assessing the degree of "faith," it is instructive also to look at the magnitude of response, as well as trends. Again the results seem equivocal. Only for three items—the item on following doctor's orders, and the two reflecting differential treatment of the elderly—did at least seven out of every ten respondents give a favorable reply. Most of the other items received only a 50 to 60 percent favorable response, while two others were under 50 percent. One of the latter, item 10, is particularly interesting because almost two-thirds of the sample gave an unfavorable response to a statement that taps a "negative" aspect of the science of medicine as contrasted with the art of medicine, namely that in their preoccupation with diagnostic gadgetry, physicians often neglect the patient as a person.

Overall, then, there seems to have been a positive change in attitudes toward physicians on specific dimensions of age-related treatment, but a decline in favorable attitude along dimensions of cost, physicians' motivations, and interest. None of the individual statements reflect very strongly held attitudes or major shifts in attitudes by this group of older respondents on any individual item.

The statements are summarized in a single index that sums each respondent's replies to all the items. These data are shown in quintile scores in Table 5.6. The general trend was toward loss of faith in physicians. Thus, there was a decline over time in the percentage of respondents who scored in the first quintile (1.80 to 1.99) and a slight increase in the percentage of those nearer the bottom, that is, holding the least favorable attitude. Although the differences are not great, the situation in 1971 did contrast somewhat with the stable response patterns of 1966 and 1968.

Changes in Definition of Health Status

The innovation of Medicare was expected to lead to higher utilization of health services, but only after a change in the definition of what constitutes an illness and for what conditions a person may legitimately seek

TABLE 5.6: Index of Faith in Physicians, Kansas City (in percent)

Index Scores	1966	1968	1971
1.80–1.99 (Favorable)	33	33	29
1.60–1.79	35	35	36
1.40–1.59	21	23	23
1.20–1.39	9	8	10
1.00–1.19 (Unfavorable)	2	1	2
N	865	705	699
Mean score	1.68	1.68	1.66

Source: Coe, et al., 1973, table IV-8.

professional services and what conditions should be dealt with in other ways. Some evidence that there was a shift in definition of illness is seen in Table 5.7. For every symptom, there was an increase from 1966 to 1971 in the percentage of respondents who claimed that they would seek a doctor's care if they had experienced the symptom. Most rapid change seems to have occurred between 1966 and 1968, with only slight change between 1968 and

TABLE 5.7: Percentage of Elderly without Symptoms Who Would Seek Physician's Care as an Initial Response if the Symptom Occurred

Symptom	1966	1968	1971
Pain in chest	72	75	83
(N)	(687)	(553)	(524)
Shortness of breath	69	75	75
(N)	(610)	(492)	(457)
Impaired hearing	75	83	84
(N)	(646)	(519)	(514)
Continued coughing	72	78	81
(N)	(782)	(649)	(629)
Pains in joints	56	55	63
(N)	(425)	(273)	(318)
Constant tiredness	61	65	66
(N)	(648)	(534)	(556)
Swelling ankles	77	78	79
(N)	(670)	(537)	(556)

Source: Coe, et al., 1973, table IV-9.

1971. Three exceptions to that pattern were pains in chest and pains in joints, which showed most change in the latter period, and swollen ankles, where the rate of increase was negligible. It should also be noted that for every symptom, a majority of respondents stated they would seek a physician's care as an initial response. Except for pains in joints and constant tiredness (often attributed to normal aging), the percentages reach 75 to 80. This very positive response is important since it contrasts sharply with the behavioral response reported by these elderly, which is discussed below.

If the data on response to hypothetical symptoms may be taken as prima-facie evidence of a change in definition of illness, one may ask about changes in perception of health status. Some data in Table 5.8 would suggest that there was no significant change in perception of health status for respondents in the three samples, although there were minor shifts within categories. It should be noted, however, that perception of health was inversely related to frequency of physician visits at a statistically significant level (p<.01). Thus, the respondent's subjective impression was still an important predictor of utilization.

Another way to view perceived health status of the elderly is according to functional ability or disability. Thus each of the surveys included the question "Do you consider yourself disabled in any way?" The percentages of respondents replying "yes" to that question were 26 in 1966, and 30 in 1968 and 1971. Thus a substantial minority of these elderly considered themselves disabled in some fashion, but the percentage increase is not impressive. A follow-up question asked in 1968 and 1971 only concerning limitation on mobility imposed by the disability showed an interesting difference in responses of workers and homemakers to that question. These data are summarized in Table 5.9. The limitations apply to the work setting for workers and retired people (nonworkers), and to the home for home-makers. The small number of respondents in the worker category report an improvement in health status; that is, few were limited. Nonworkers show no

TABLE 5.8:   Perceived Health Status of the Elderly (in percent)

Perceived health status	1965	1968	1971
Excellent	30	28	26
Good	31	33	36
Fair	26	25	27
Poor	13	15	11
Total	100	100	100
N	870	705	700

Source: Coe, et al., 1973, table IV-2.

TABLE 5.9: **Perceived Limitations by Respondents with Disabilities (in percent)**

	Workers		Nonworkers		Homemakers	
Degree of Limitations	1968	1971	1968	1971	1968	1971
Severe limitation	6	–	7	7	8	18
Some limitation	75	74	84	87	86	89
No limitation	18	26	9	6	7	3
Total	100	100	100	100	100	100
N	17	19	98	124	248	76

Source: Compiled by the authors.

change, and homemakers show a decline in health status; that is, more were limited. The reasons for this difference in responses are not clear.

In summary, then, the Medicare program seems to have contributed to a broadened definition of illness by the elderly. At the same time, there was very little shift in perception of health status or of limitations imposed by any form of disability.

Changing the Sick Role

At the very least, one can conclude that there was considerable illness among the respondents of this study. Except for continued coughing, more than one-fifth reported experiencing each of the other symptoms, although there is no apparent relationship between degree of seriousness and frequency of experience. Thus, there seems to be increased opportunity to evaluate other aspects of illness-related behavior. Perhaps most crucial in this respect is the initial response to the symptoms. These data for those who experienced the symptom are shown in Part A of Table 5.10. Also included for comparison purposes are data concerning the proportion who *ever* saw a physician for the symptom (Part B) and the percentage who said they would seek a physician's care first if they ever had the symptom (Part C).

There are several notable features of the data in Table 5.10. First is an apparently consistent pattern, at least with respect to differences between 1968 and 1971, of what the respondent would do first. Except for swollen ankles, fewer respondents waited to see if the symptom would go away— more so for continued coughing, constant tiredness, and impaired hearing than for other symptoms. For shortness of breath (a serious symptom) the change was to taking medicine already on hand. Otherwise, for the most serious symptoms, more people went to the physician as the initial response, while taking medicine on hand was the main change for minor symptoms, with a decline in choosing to go to the physician first. This was especially the case for swelling ankles.

TABLE 5.10: Initial Response to Symptom Experience, by Symptom (in percent)

	Pain in Chest			Shortness of Breath			Impaired Hearing			Continued Coughing			Pains in Joints			Constant Tiredness			Swelling Ankles		
	1966	1968	1971	1966	1968	1971	1966	1968	1971	1966	1968	1971	1966	1968	1971	1966	1968	1971	1966	1968	1971
A. Initial Response																					
Wait, do nothing	27	28	24	44	54	41	50	55	47	30	40	29	27	28	22	47	46	38	37	31	33
Take medicine	33	34	32	22	11	18	3	3	2	38	24	30	37	36	41	22	16	17	23	23	29
See doctor right away	40	38	43	43	32	39	43	32	39	33	31	40	35	34	33	30	34	32	41	44	34
Other	—	—	1	—	2	7	2	10	11	—	5	1	1	2	4	1	5	13	—	2	4
N	181	152	176	255	211	242	203	186	184	80	55	70	438	432	381	218	171	204	194	167	144
B. See doctor at all? (percent of respondents saying yes)	76	78	81	69	61	71	57	54	58	66	63	66	72	69	69	59	61	65	74	72	74
N	687	553	524	610	492	457	646	519	514	782	649	629	425	273	318	648	534	496	670	537	556
C. Percent who would see doctor first if had symptom	72	75	83	69	75	75	75	83	84	72	78	81	56	55	63	61	65	66	77	78	79
N	687	553	524	610	492	457	646	519	514	782	649	629	425	273	318	648	534	496	670	537	556

— = less than 1 percent.

Source: Coe, et al., 1973, Table N-12.

A second change—related to the first—is the relative frequency of choosing a physician as a first response. Theoretically, physician's services should be sought first for the most serious symptoms. In 1971, this would seem to be the case for the four most serious symptoms. But this represented a considerable shift since 1968, when physician services were sought first most often for the least serious symptoms, except for pains in the chest. In part, this change may reflect the increased reported prevalence of the serious symptoms in 1971. However, it may also represent a change in norms relating to seeking professional care, *but more oriented to acute symptomatology than to an orientation to care of chronic illnesses*. That is, seeking a physician's care as an initial response increased most for pains in chest, continued coughing, and impaired hearing. This interpretation is supported also by the responses of respondents who had not experienced those symptoms. That is, most said that *if* they had chest pains, shortness of breath, and so on, they would go first to a physician (see Part C of Table 5.10). For every symptom, the percentage responding this way equaled or exceeded the percentage in 1968. Most notable of all, however, is the consistent and significant discrepancy between those with symptoms who actually went first to a physician and those without symptoms who stated they would go first to a physician.

There is some evidence, however, that counters that interpretation, namely, the proportion who *ever* saw a physician for an episode of the symptom (see Part B, Table 5.10). For every symptom, there was a substantial increase in the percentage of respondents who eventually saw a physician. In most cases, at least 20 percent more respondents saw a doctor in 1971 than in 1968 for any given symptom. It may also be seen that the major stimuli to seeking care are *pain* (pain in chest, pain in joints and muscles) and *interference with normal activities* (caused by swelling ankles and shortness of breath). It may be, then, that the *pattern* of response did not change, but the *level* of seeking professional care increased markedly. This would suggest that there was some change in what is defined as "illness" for which it is appropriate to seek professional care. The data presented in Table 5.11 on the *length of delay* in seeking a doctor's care also relate to the question of whether a normative shift took place. These data indicate that between 1968 and 1971 the basic pattern showed either a reduced percentage waiting one month or longer to seek care, or an increase in the percentage of those who waited one week or less. This would imply a normative shift occurred. However, if the entire time period is considered, a different picture emerges. The pattern then appears to be an initial increase in delay in seeking a physician's care, with a later shift to reduced delay. The later shift did not equal the initial increase in delay, so that the net result over the time period was for greater delay in seeking a physician's care. The difference in time pattern between the first years and 1968 to 1971 is similar to what was seen in the discussion of changes in the average number of physician visits. It

TABLE 5.11: Delay in Seeking a Physician's Care, by Symptom, 1966, 1968, and 1971 (percent)

Length of Delay	Pain in Chest 1966	1968	1971	Shortness of Breath 1966	1968	1971	Impaired Hearing 1966	1968	1971	Continued Coughing 1966	1968	1971	Pains in Joints 1966	1968	1971	Constant Tiredness 1966	1968	1971	Swelling Ankles 1966	1968	1971
Less than or equal to 1 week	74	60	63	62	54	62	38	36	40	71	53	56	74	44	46	47	40	52	54	53	50
More than one week, but less than or equal to 1 month	15	21	25	21	22	23	27	33	26	13	24	20	17	21	22	29	28	26	28	20	21
More than 1 month	8	17	11	12	21	14	26	25	32	8	21	24	4	31	30	18	31	22	14	23	27
Other or don't know	3	2	1	6	3	2	9	6	2	8	3	—	4	5	2	5	—	1	4	4	2
N	123	117	143	159	125	171	117	84	106	24	34	46	69	283	298	99	106	133	125	115	105

— = less than 1 percent.

Source: Coe, et al., 1973, Table IV-13.

is interesting that delay shifts affected the most-serious as well as the least-serious symptoms. It would be difficult to evaluate this movement over time as a normative shift, although viewing the later short-term situation provides some support for this contention.

UTILIZATION AND COST OF HEALTH CARE SERVICES

This section reports data from a series of questions on physician visits, hospitalizations, and the noninsured costs of medical services for older persons. The data reviewed in Chapter 4 are National Health Survey data or are related to program use and costs. These data are from the interviews with elderly persons in Kansas City only.

Physician Visits

Questions concerning physician visits in 1968 and 1971 excluded doctor's visits in hospitals and nursing homes. Since the wording of this question included hospitals and nursing homes in 1966, the 1966 data are not comparable.

As Table 5.12 shows, the median number of visits to physicians increased from 2.8 per year in 1968 to 3.4 per year in 1971. The percent who did not visit physicians at all and the percent with relatively few (1 to 3) visits declined, while the percent with 4 to 10 visits per year increased from 23 percent to 28 percent.

The increase in physician's visits from 1968 to 1971 parallels the increase shown by the National Health Survey for that short period. The rates are not directly comparable, inasmuch as the National Health Survey includes physician visits in hospitals and utilizes a different age breakdown.

TABLE 5.12: Physician Visits per Year, 1968 and 1971 (percent distribution and median number)

Number of Visits	1968	1971
0	29	26
1–3	34	30
4–10	23	28
11 or more	13	14
Total	100	100
N	703	700
Median number of visits	2.8	3.4

Source: Coe, et al., 1973, Table IV-15.

The National Health Survey showed that the number of physician visits per person per year increased from 5.6 in 1968 to 6.4 in 1971 for the population 65–74 years of age, and from 5.9 to 7.2 for the population 75 and over (NCHS, 1968 and 1971). As reported in Chapter 4, physician use fluctuated over the years, showing an initial decrease from before to shortly after Medicare started, then an increase by 1971 to the approximate pre-Medicare level, and no basic change after that time. The Kansas City data reflect the same pattern from 1968 to 1971.

The increase from 1968 to 1971 would have generally confirmed the hypothesis that Medicare would bring about an increase in utilization of health services. However, it was not sustained in the national use data, and basically represents a return to the pre-Medicare pattern after an unexplained initial decrease in physician use.

The Kansas City data for this time period reflect changes in relative utilization among income groups. Physician visits by those who perceived their income as adequate for the Kansas City sample are shown in Table 5.13. Differences among income categories were not significant in 1968 ($p<.90$), but were in 1971 ($p<.01$). Physician visits definitely increased for the older population with inadequate incomes. Thus, in accordance with one of the purposes of the Medicare legislation, the lower-income population, which is also less healthy, was receiving more services from physicians.

Within all three samples (1966, 1968, and 1971), there were significant relationships between physician visits and health status ($p<.01$), and between physician visits and preventive care orientations ($p<.01$). In other words, those in poorer health and those oriented toward preventive care did make more use of physicians. There is no evidence in the data, however, that the increased financing of medical care produced anything that might be described as overutilization.

Hospitalization

There was no major increase reported in the proportion hospitalized during the years from 1966 (17 percent) to 1968 (20 percent) to 1971 (18 percent). Although not statistically significant, those with inadequate income reported a steady increase—from 20 percent in 1966, to 21 percent in 1968, to 24 percent in 1971. Older persons in poor health reported a major increase in hospitalization use, from 29 percent in 1966, to 39 percent in 1968, and a small decrease, to 37 percent, in 1971. As in the case of physician's visits, the effect of Medicare has been to increase utilization for the poor and for those in poor health.

For those who were hospitalized during the previous year, the total number of days of hospitalization increased. These data, based on the question, "How many nights were you in the hospital?" are shown in Table 5.14. The major increase in days of hospitalization occurred from 1968 to

TABLE 5.13: Physician Visits per Year, by Perceived Income Adequacy, 1968 and 1971 (percent distribution and median number)

Number of Physician Visits	1968			1971		
	Inadequate	Adequate	Comfortable	Inadequate	Adequate	Comfortable
0	31	29	29	27	26	26
1–3	27	31	39	19	26	38
4–10	24	23	23	29	28	27
11 or more	16	17	9	22	16	10
Total	100	100	100	100	100	100
N	97	303	302	96	295	306
Median number of visits	3.1	3.0	2.6	4.9	3.8	2.9

Source: Coe, et al., 1973, Table IV-16.

TABLE 5.14: Nights in the Hospital Reported by Those Hospitalized, 1966, 1968, and 1971 (percent distribution)

Number of Nights	1966	1968	1971
1–5	31	31	17
6–10	25	26	34
11 and over	44	43	49

Source: Coe, et al., 1973, Table IV-17.

1971. Although the subsamples become small (less than 50) when divided by income adequacy and health status, the increase in days of hospitalization seems to have occurred for all income levels and for all health status groups.

It should be noted that the increase in days of hospitalization in Kansas City is different from 1968–71 trends reported in the National Health Survey. The National Health Survey reports a decline in days of hospitalization per person from 19.3 in 1968 to 17.5 in 1971. The Kansas City data from interviews with the older population, however, do agree with other information on the decline from 1968 to 1971 in the utilization of extended care facilities and home health services.

Expenses Not Covered by Medicare and Other Insurance

In the 1966 survey, 63 percent of respondents reported medical expenses not covered by Medicare or other insurance; in the 1968 survey, 67 percent; and in 1971, 60 percent. Thus, the overall trend seems to have been toward a lowering of these figures. However, as shown in Table 5.15, of those having additional expenses, the proportion of those paying higher amounts increased. This is in keeping with general increases in the cost of medical services.

TABLE 5.15: Medical Bills Not Covered by Medicare or Other Insurance (percent distribution by amount for those incurring bills)

Amount of Bills	1966	1968	1971
Under $50	23	19	11
$50–99	16	22	19
$100–199	20	23	28
$200–299	10	14	12
$300 and over	20	22	30

Source: Coe, et al., 1973, Table IV-18.

Table 5.16 shows the source of funds for medical bills not covered by Medicare or other insurance. In interpreting the table, it should be kept in mind that respondents do not necessarily differentiate between Medicare and Medicaid. However, there seems to be a pronounced decline in "bills not paid." Certainly most such payments continued to derive from the patient's own resources.

Finally, in connection with medical expenses not covered by Medicare or other insurance, patients were asked, "As a result of your expenses, did you put off any medical treatment . . . buying anything you needed, trips or vacation . . . anything else?" As shown in Table 5.17, all such effects consistently increased in importance from 1966 to 1968 to 1971. Doubtless, such consequences reflect the increase in the amount of uncovered bills (shown in Table 5.15).

Perception of Community's Health System

We have seen that Medicare had some impact on the elderly in terms of changes in definitions of illness, but less influence on their illness-related behavior. Now we wish to examine the perceptions of the consumers with respect to Medicare's effects on the health services in their community. It was hypothesized that the elderly would become increasingly critical of health services even though still mostly positive as most laymen are. This is because Medicare held out a promise that raised expectations of the elderly that were not, and probably could not be, fulfilled completely under the present system. Some clue to the relationship between a change in perceptions, with a lack of change in behavior of the elderly and a lack of actual change in organization of health services, may be found in the perception of the elderly of their community's health services.

One of the general questions asked in 1968 and 1971 concerned perception of the quality of care by doctors. As expected, the response was overwhelmingly favorable, but between 1968 and 1971 showed a decline in favorable response. In 1968, 95 percent rated the quality of physician care as

TABLE 5.16: Source of Funds for Medical Bills Not Covered by Medicare or Other Insurance (percent distribution of those incurring bills)

Source of Funds	1966	1968	1971
Own resources	89	97	95
Relatives	3	1	3
Welfare	2	1	1
Bills not paid	6	1	1

Source: Coe, et al., 1973, table IV-19.

TABLE 5.17:   Some Effects of Medical Expenses Not Covered by Medicare or Other Insurance (percent distribution of those incurring bills)

Effect	1966	1968	1971
Put off medical treatment	8	10	14
Put off buying something needed	24	25	33
Put off trip or vacation	17	18	23
Put off other expenses	6	15	17

Note: Because the questions were asked individually, they do not add up to 100 percent.
Source: Coe, et al., 1973, Table IV-20.

excellent or good (N=634). In the follow-up in 1971, the same responses were given by 88 percent (N=639). In effect, there remained a considerable degree of confidence in physician's services. The specific effect of Medicare on physicians' willingness to serve the elderly is suggested in Table 5.18. The response is positive, although the shift is not statistically significant in magnitude (p.<.10). There is, however, an important decline from 1968 to 1971 in the proportion of the total sample who had no opinion.

Respondents were then asked if their community had the type of health services they might need. The responses were generally positive, but again showed a decline from 1968 to 1971. In the first period, 81 percent responded positively to the question. In 1971, the percentage had dropped to 75 percent, still a substantial majority. One follow-up question asked if the

TABLE 5.18:   Perception by Elderly of Physicians' Attention to Problems of People over Age 60 since Medicare (in percent)

Degree of Attention	1968	1971
More	14.6	20.2
Same	78.1	72.7
Less	7.3	7.1
Total	100.0	100.0
N	479 (67.9)	554 (79.1)
Don't know	226 (32.1)	146 (20.9)
Total N	705 (100.0)	700 (100.0)

Source: Compiled by the authors.

respondent had wanted to see a physician, but could not, and if so, why not. Only 12.5 percent (N=87) stated this had happened to them in 1971. The reasons most frequently cited were: (1) the visit would have been too expensive (37 percent); (2) no transportation was available (31 percent); (3) respondent was physically unable (16 percent); and (4) doctors were not available (15 percent). This small subsample reported some barriers to receiving care that relate directly to problems the Medicare program was intended to ease.

In regard to the provision of health services in the community, all respondents were asked what could be done to improve the health care for people over age 60. Their responses are shown in Table 5.19. First, it should be noted that between 1968 and 1971 there was a substantial increase in the proportion of respondents who felt that something more was needed, and a decline in the percentage of those who either did not know what more could be done or who felt that the system was adequate as it was.

Secondly, it appears that in 1968 the major concern was with availability, the physical presence of personnel and facilities. In 1971, except for a perceived need for more physicians, perceived needs shifted to more ambulatory clinics and transportation, that is, accessibility to health care resources. This interpretation supports the perceptions of respondents who had wanted to see a physician, but could not because doctors were unavailable or because the respondents could not get to them.

Another way to look at these data is in terms of the implicit and explicit intent of the Medicare legislation. Some of the expressed needs reflect the concepts of accountability for and acceptability of health services also. Of the 18 items in Table 5.19, 7 are directly related to health. These address the issue of availability and express a need for more personnel and/or facilities. Of these, the need for more physicians and more clinics showed significant increases in priority from 1968 to 1971. The perception of the need for other personnel changed very little or actually decreased in priority.

Two items refer explicitly to accessibility: increased access to doctors and adequate transportation. Both show sharp increases from 1968 to 1971 and were high-priority items as well. It must be concluded, therefore, that the implicit intent of Medicare to improve availability and accessibility of health services through better organization of community health resources was not fulfilled, as perceived by consumers. In view of the discussion in Chapter 4 about the failure to obtain any reorganization, the perceptions of the elderly consumer seem very appropriate.

Four of the items refer to the concept of affordability or increased ability to purchase services. None of these items was very frequently cited and the degree of change from 1968 to 1971 was negligible. Only for "lower physician's charges" was the percentage change large, but the number of people involved was less than 7 percent of the total.

The two remaining concepts descriptive of health services, accountabil-

TABLE 5.19: Perception by the Elderly of Changes Necessary for Improving Community Health Services (in percent)

Perceived Need	1968	1971
More doctors	17.3	23.2
More hospitals	10.8	6.7
More nurses	8.7	5.5
Increased access to doctors	8.7	16.8
Improvement in hospitals	8.7	1.8
Cheaper nursing homes	8.7	9.4
More clinics	6.5	13.8
More home visiting nurses	6.5	6.7
Better-equipped nursing homes	6.5	12.0
Someone to help the aged	6.5	3.0
More nursing homes	4.3	4.1
More inspected nursing homes	4.3	3.9
Lower physician's charges	4.3	6.9
Government help with medical care	4.3	2.8
Increased social security	4.3	2.5
Cheaper housing	4.3	4.6
More income	2.2	1.4
Better-qualified help	2.2	0.9
Adequate transportation	2.2	12.9
Medical supervision	2.2	—
More activities for the aged	2.2	2.8
More dentists	—	1.6
Better politicians	2.2	0.9
All other	13.0	12.7
N	323 (46.0)	434 (62.2)
Nothing is needed	154 (21.9)	108 (15.5)
Don't know	224 (32.1)	156 (22.3)
Totals	702 (100.0)	698 (100.0)

Note: Totals do not equal 100 percent since some respondents made more than one response.

Source: Compiled by the authors.

ity and acceptability, were not high-priority items, but the shifts in perceptions are interesting. Accountability refers to quality of care rendered and who is responsible for monitoring it. All four items referring to accountability (nursing home inspections, hospital improvement, medical supervision, and better-qualified help) show *decreases* from 1968 to 1971 in percentage of respondents citing them. The high priority of the issue of mechanisms of accountability in professional circles is not shared by these consumers. Only one item, better-equipped nursing homes, seems to reflect consumer acceptability, and this showed a strong positive change from 1968 to 1971.

SUMMARY: THE IMPACT OF MEDICARE FOR
THE OLDER POPULATION

On the whole, the effect of the Medicare program on and for the older population was less than we anticipated. Physician visits increased from 1968 to 1971 for the older population in Kansas City, and most of this was increased utilization by those who reported their income as inadequate and by those in poor health. Those poorer in income, health, or both also reported an increase in hospitalization from 1966 to 1971. Thus, the major effect appears to have been to increase the affordability of and accessibility to health services for the disadvantaged.

There is no indication in the data of overutilization of services on the part of older consumers. To the extent that overutilization may have occurred, it is reflected in an increase in days of hospitalization in Kansas City from 1968 to 1971, as reported by older respondents. In other sections, we have discussed the failure to develop home health services and extended care facilities as an alternate to hospitalization. The failure to utilize such alternatives is, of course, beyond the control of consumers.

Increased ability to pay for services did not increase satisfaction with services. The attitudes of the noninstitutionalized older population toward nursing homes remained very negative. Confidence in physicians and in hospitals was relatively higher, yet composite indexes of attitudes toward physicians, hospitals, and nursing homes showed some decline by 1971, partly due to increased concern about costs.

Increased concern about the costs of services was reflected in several parts of the interview. About one-eighth of the total sample reported that they had wanted to see a doctor but could not, because the visit would have been too expensive, or because they had no transportation (which is related to cost). The size of bills not covered by Medicare or other insurance increased considerably from 1968 to 1971. Because of such bills, more respondents reported they had put off medical treatment and other purchases.

The expectation that Medicare might affect the normative orientation toward illness was not generally confirmed. Respondents showed some increased inclination to seek assistance for symptoms encountered and to seek such assistance earlier. There was also a slight increase in those reporting a preventive-care orientation. On the whole, however, there appears to be little change in the health-seeking orientation of the older population.

Our data suggest that, from the perspective of the elderly consumer, Medicare influenced the definition of illness and, perhaps, altered public expectations of what the community's health care system would provide. Independently, we noted that the program's implicit intent to create a better organization of services was not accomplished, and that this fact is reflected in the perception of the elderly citizens. They reported a positive attitude toward doctors in the community, but decreased availability and accessibility of services. In the absence of any effective organization or even coordination of health resources, the increased demand by the elderly as part of the change in expectation created more severe problems in the delivery system. This was accurately perceived by the elderly, and these concerns replaced problems of financing health care. This explicit aim of the program was met at least to the extent that costs of services were less a priority than their availability or accessibility.

6
CONCLUSIONS AND IMPLICATIONS

This book has examined the problem of the health care needs of the aged as this one aspect of the broader issue of national policy on health and health care of the population was uniquely approached in the United States.

The social value traditions underlying health care, social insurance, and social welfare set the parameters within which any effort to deal with the health care needs of the aged could be considered. At the time the Medicare and Medicaid amendments were passed, it would not have been possible to establish a consensus on an overall national health policy or even on a broad policy for the health of the aged. Establishing a policy of financing health services for the aged in relation to health care as a right and not a privilege was itself a major accomplishment.

PROBLEM, POLICY, AND PROGRAM: CASE OF THE IMPERFECT FIT

The general thesis, as stated before, is that failure of a program to solve a recognized problem may result from an "imperfect fit" between the definition of a problem and the policy articulated to deal with the problem, or between the intent of a policy—that is, the approach to the problem—and the design and implementation of the program developed to carry out the intent. This may result in a mismatch between the program and the underlying problem. In the present case, health care needs of the aged, the nature and scope of the problem were too narrowly identified in the process of policy formulation. Subsequently, the legislated program that emerged bore characteristics that made its "fit" to intent of the policy less than perfect.

With respect to problem definition, the problem was too narrowly defined. There was a failure to consider the nature of the problem in the context of multiproblem, elderly families. Despite significant evidence that the problem was not solely one of the economics of health care for the aged, the policy underlying the Medicare program focused on the ability to pay for that care as the issue of concern. Other, peripheral aspects of the problem of the health of the aged were not considered. It is in this sense that we refer to the policy toward dealing with the financing of health care for the aged through Medicare as a mismatch or "imperfect fit" to the underlying problem of the health needs of the aged.

Once defined from this perspective, the problem of health care for the aged was more easily addressed as a separate entity, rather than as part of any effort to deal with the more general issues of health care delivery and financing for the entire population, which have been dealt with in other developed countries.

When unmet health needs were at last seen as a problem, the initial answers to what should be done ranged from development of a reorganized, comprehensive health system to "doing nothing" because the elderly "preferred to disengage." Under this latter assumption, health care and other support services were neither necessary nor wanted. As we have seen, however, the problem was defined in terms of inability to pay for medical services; thus, a program needed only to provide funds to purchase services. Though political trade-offs were involved in the narrow way the problem was defined, the definition arrived at was consistent with an American perspective on market mechanisms in which an infusion of money produces "ripple" effects. Given our current knowledge of the many-faceted nature of the problem of the health of the elderly, the decision to focus on the financial barriers to care alone was inappropriate.

With this definition, the question of concern for our analysis then became, How well did the Medicare program serve the policy goals for which it was instituted? Policy development on the issue of lowering financial barriers was complicated by consideration of personal versus public responsibility for the situation of the aged. Public responsibility was acknowledged, at least in part, for the low-income status of the elderly, but there was no acceptance of responsibility for the health care system by public leaders, and certainly no one was responsible for aging. Thus, public sources might be used for financially aiding the elderly; reorganizing the system, however, was not then considered part of the matter under consideration.

With an imperfect fit between the underlying problem and the policy formulated to deal with it, the Medicare program itself had at least three major conceptual difficulties as a vehicle for carrying out even the policy as developed.

First, the program did not affect the autonomy of the medical profession. Although physicians were seen as the key to use of a community's health system, there was an explicit disavowal of any "interference with the practice of medicine." Thus, measures intended to change ways doctors used the system or to create viable alternatives to traditional acute-care resources were bound to fail.

Second, the program did not include cost-efficiency incentives for providers. Rapidly rising costs of the program, especially for hospital care, have continued to be a major concern. Yet initially, providers were to be reimbursed on a "cost-plus" basis, that is, payment of approved costs plus a small overhead. Later, this became a cost-only reimbursement (and not total costs). At no time, however, has policy ever included incentives to encourage providers to be more economically efficient or to encourage their cooperative organization (Feder, 1977). As a result, the traditional competition for more services and expensive technology among institutional providers in a community continues unabated. The major difference is the number of federal dollars that feeds the competition.

Third, the program misapplied the concept of "spell of illness." Adoption of a concept that bore little relevance to the recognized nature of the health problems of the aged undermined the potential for achieving even the explicit intent of the program, i.e., to reduce the financial barriers to care for the elderly. Instead of a concept of health maintenance or surveillance, which implies frequent and regular utilization of health services (not necessarily a physician), the policy makers adopted the concept of "spell of illness," more relevant to acute-care, crisis-oriented medicine.

The data we have presented strongly suggest that the Medicare program, despite some areas of specific accomplishment, did not adequately carry out the explicit intent to reduce the financial barriers to health care among the aged. The level of out-of-pocket expenditures for health care by the aged was reduced only marginally in comparison with the major increases in total costs and public expenditures for health care. Additionally, the design and operation of the program itself were probably major factors in the failure to provide incentives for the development of alternatives to the most expensive form of medical service, in-patient hospital care. Finally, there was no appreciable reorganization of the medical care delivery system to make it more responsive to the unique health needs of the aged, which we have called the implicit intent of Medicare. It is in this sense that we conclude that the Medicare program, as passed and implemented, was a mismatch to the policy it was developed to carry out.

The two major areas of change were discussed relative to medical care delivery before and after Medicare: patterns of use and cost. The program design seems to have encouraged an increase in the use of in-patient hospital care as contrasted to ambulatory care. While the short-stay hospital admission rate increased over time, and more out of every 1,000 older persons were being served by the hospital in-patient reimbursement portion of the program, the average length of stay was reduced, so that days of care per 1,000 older persons did not increase. With more older persons hospitalized for shorter average lengths of stay, the possibility has to be considered that there may be more hospitalizations for less serious issues among aged patients. It may be that advances in medical care technology and procedures have shortened the time these patients need the intensity of care available only in the hospital setting. If either or a combination of these possibilities is the case, then the failure to develop the skilled nursing facility/extended care facility may be extracting a very high price in both program dollars and the inappropriate use of in-patient hospital beds. The most extreme form of such a situation would be the use of a short-stay hospital bed for the long-term hospitalization of an aged patient because an SNF is not available.

Reimbursement policy and the use of deductibles and co-insurance, commonly associated with illness insurance, limited rather than stimulated utilization of the less expensive forms of care. More recent rises in amount of liability to enrollees has reached the point where even needed acute care will be difficult for the elderly to obtain, thus tarnishing the one positive contribution of the program to health care for the elderly. The absolute number of out-of-pocket dollars and the percent of retirement benefits used for medical care for the aged now as compared to before Medicare further exacerbate the problem.

The combination of increased use of hospital care and inflation in unit cost has resulted in tremendously higher overall program costs for in-patient care in more recent years than at the start of the program. While program costs for ambulatory care have increased, these have not gone up at anything approaching the rate of increase for in-patient care. The overall result is that the total costs for the Medicare program went up more rapidly than anticipated. The ability to rationalize the use of medical care services and to influence the patterns of care in favor of less expensive and possibly more appropriate forms of care through adjustment of reimbursement mechanisms or direct control over aspects of the delivery system itself could have a significant effect on medical care expenditures in the future for the aged. Can the "imperfect fit" between problem and policy and between policy and program be made more perfect? It seems altogether possible, especially if one observes the approaches taken to health care for the elderly, indeed for whole populations, in other countries. Additionally, the experience under Medicare strongly suggests the degree to which patterns of medical care may be alterable. It seems clear also that continued "tinkering" with the program through minor adjustments of reimbursement policy, eligibility, coverage, and even incentives for more economical use will not affect much the imperfect fit (Weil, 1976).

Health Status of the Elderly

Aside from the possible effect of Medicare on the use, cost, and delivery of health services for the aged, medical services alone did not make any improvement in the health status of the elderly. That is, provision of physicians' services, hospital care, home health services and nursing home care, and limited guarantees of payment for care did not result in measurable improvement in the indicators of health status. Studies of the "situation" of the elderly in communities and institutions still reveal an alarming picture (cf. the review in Shanas and Maddox, 1976). For example, life expectancy at age 65 or older has not improved for white males, and only small gains have been observed for white females and for nonwhites of both sexes. Rates of mortality have always been highest for the elderly, and the rate is still ten times higher than the average for all age groups. The major causes of death continue to be heart disease, cancer, and stroke. Rates of morbidity show excessive prevalence of chronic diseases among the elderly, but lower incidence of acute disorders than among younger age groups. The degree of impairment and resulting limitation of activities are higher among older people than younger ones.

Surveys of the elderly report that their perceived health status, as contrasted with objective, physical examination findings, tends to be over-estimated by the elderly and highly related to symptoms that interfere with normal activities (Larson, 1978). Thus, the elderly correctly perceive their needs in terms of care for chronic, impairing health problems. These types of problems require frequent monitoring, but little technical skill by health providers, to limit, if not prevent, the disability associated with impairment.

Over and above the issue of the effect on their health status, the elderly continue to perceive problems with meeting their health needs that are independent of the financing issue. These difficulties relate to long waits for appointments with physicians, and problems with transportation. Scheduling appointments is more problematic as demand for physicians' services increases. Most elderly live in urban areas, but in the older parts of the city, while hospitals and physicians' offices are found primarily in suburban areas. Thus, transportation to services is an additional problem. For the substantial proportion of elderly in some rural areas and small towns, accessibility to services is even more reduced.

PERSPECTIVES ON THE HEALTH CARE SYSTEM

The prevailing pattern of organization of health services in U.S. communities is important to consider in any attempt to analyze the impact of Medicare on the health care delivery system. The general hospital has served as the focus of health services. Much emphasis is placed on in-patient care, although most doctors who practice in the general hospital are in private practice and collect fees for services they provide both in the hospital and in their own offices. Over the years, a number of agencies have developed that provide additional health services for various population groups. To the extent that service providers are associated, it has been largely through limited referral networks, usually with the physician as the central organizing point and seldom with either the "package" of services or the consumer as the core concern (Coe et al., 1974).

Medicare was expected to encourage greater diversity in care for the elderly through a transitional, less expensive form of in-patient care, that is, the ECF, in combination with care for the ambulatory in their own homes (home health services); promote continuity by connecting various types of services to provide comprehensive care; and facilitate the implementation of preventive care and health maintenance, including a system of regular continuing contact between older patients and comprehensive health services.

Medicare did not have the effect expected. Moreover, Medicare, by itself and in its present form, will probably not have a substantial effect on the organization of health care services or on patterns of use in the older population.

We have noted that Medicare was a new payment program for health services and have described the antecedent conditions leading to the emergence of the program as a compromise response. One way to consider the outcome of this program is to examine its acceptance by or integration into society. Acceptance depends in part upon the program's demonstrating of its superiority over what it replaces. In these terms, the Medicare program may be judged superior to what it replaced. It increased the access of older persons, especially the disadvantaged, to health services they needed. It also reduced the potential depletion of their assets by the need for prolonged medical care.

Most of the Kansas City physicians interviewed, and those from other studies (Coe and Sigler, 1970; Colombotos, 1968, 1969) supported Medicare as an insurance mechanism, although some reservations were expressed about "long-term effects." Certainly many physicians have benefited financially from the program because of the provisions of the legislation. The existing health care delivery system received increased financial support from the program. One of the elements of the failure of the Medicare program to have the far-reaching effects predicted for it was that physicians remained in control of the network of services. Their position probably was strengthened by the increased number and level of services under Medicare. As presently designed, the program in no way penalizes physicians for not making changes in the system or in their practices. Hospital use by the doctor is rewarded both professionally and economically. Other levels of care can be used, but usually only if the hospital's needs for full beds are satisfied. The relationship of nursing homes to hospitals is largely confined to referral. In general, physicians relate infrequently and almost tangentially to nursing homes or patients in these homes.

If the health delivery system is to be encouraged to change to serve the needs of the aged more effectively, rewards have to be provided for such change. What is required is change in the program and in reimbursement practices, combined with general efforts to encourage the development of comprehensive, coordinated health care delivery systems.

Legislative proposals have been introduced periodically for some form of national health insurance for the entire population. The current proposals that realistically could be approved by Congress would not be an effective approach to the problem (Bodenheimer, 1972). Indeed, they may only extend to the entire population the current difficulties of providing care discussed here. Experience under the Medicare program can provide insights applicable to future efforts. One principle that should be included in any new legislation is to incorporate incentives for providers to change the health care delivery system. In the long view, changes in conceptualization of the problem and ethical perspectives on resource allocation to meet the problem must precede more extensive systemic changes in delivery of health services.

IMPLICATIONS FOR PROGRAM DEVELOPMENT

Against the background of this review of Medicare and its impact, we need to look to recommendations for its alteration and possible approaches to be taken to health services for the aged in particular and to health care in general. Some mechanisms for getting where we want to go are short-range and involve the immediate program; others are longer-range and involve a more general national health policy.

It should be abundantly clear that we believe that in a broad sense the Medicare program has failed to alter significantly the health care situation for the elderly. This does not deny that some temporary improvements were made in reducing economic barriers to care and in creating new resources for health care. Our global judgment is based on the lack of a system focus on the initial problem and the consequent piecemeal programmatic attack on the problem. In our evaluation, several major factors underlying the health care needs of the population were pointed out along with the obvious conclusion that resolving the problem would mean dealing with most of these factors simultaneously.

The importance of a more comprehensive approach to developing an effective health delivery system is increased now because of the current push for some form of national health insurance or a similar program that would provide insurance against sickness for the whole population and not just the elderly. There is also talk of increasing benefits beyond current levels of Medicare. Given the rapidly escalating costs of even the present limited Medicare program, the costs for a similar program for the other 89 percent of the population could be astronomical. Therefore, alternatives to the present system must be developed. To facilitate a brief discussion of the issues, it is helpful to return to the paradigm of five *a*'s (availability, accessibility, affordability, accountability, and acceptability). These help us to determine some elements of a national health policy, but from a system perspective.

It should be remembered that *availability* refers to the presence of a range of health professionals in sufficient numbers. This implies some balance between primary care and other specialties among physicians, as well as adequate numbers of nurses, social workers, and other allied health professionals. *Accessibility* to these personnel is a different but equally important dimension that refers to their distribution in the population. *Affordability*, of course, relates to ability to pay for services used and is the dimension of principal concern to the present Medicare program. *Accountability* describes the need for providers to be responsible for the quality of services rendered, including a dimension of comprehensiveness through co-ordination. Patient satisfaction with services received, including consideration of the patient's dignity as a person, underlies the variable of *acceptability*.

One specific recommendation that relates to the current Medicare program, but also has implications for any more comprehensive program effort, is that, at a minimum, the bias in favor of reimbursement for in-patient care as compared with ambulatory care should be altered. The intent may well have related to a concern for the potential impact of an actual or projected hospital bill of major proportions on the financial situation of an aged person, or the use of these services among the aged. However, the imbalance in reimbursement policy seems to have provided a spur to use of in-patient care. It would be far more appropriate from an economic and resource-allocation perspective to reinforce use of the least expensive form of care suitable to the needs of the situation. While discouraging hospital use when needed is not the intent, the experience of various health maintenance organizations in controlling in-patient care attests to the potential for the use of financial incentives for influencing use patterns.

An approach of this nature is a means of using financial incentives to influence care patterns. It is a recognition of the fact that any reimbursement mechanism may affect the use of services in ways related to the program's design features. An alternative, and more direct, approach to controlling care patterns is to establish a framework of care standards. Such standards can be used to assure, from two perspectives, the quality of care delivered. First, the care delivered must meet certain standards of quality, and, second, the use of services should not be beyond the requirements of the situation when more appropriate care is available. Efforts to accomplish the second purpose are included in various Medicare provisions, such as the use of utilization review committees. However, these have not been overwhelmingly effective. The specter of control over the system for delivery of health care and for establishing enforceable standards for quality of care gave rise to Section 1801 of the Social Security Act as amended in 1965.

The general direction in which we should be heading in any effort to reconsider our program directions or to determine an appropriate national health policy has been suggested previously:

> Since a considerable amount of research has shown time and again that our present fee-for-service organization of medicine is dysfunctional in terms of providing certain groups with adequate medical care—especially the poor and the aged—it would seem reasonable that some form of subsidized care would be provided. Medicare and Medicaid, of course, already provide some precedent for this approach. But these programs are not oriented to altering the present system for delivery of medical care. They provide financial support for the present system of delivery which is oriented primarily toward dealing with illness, not promoting health. What is needed is a combination of subsidized care and a reorientation of the delivery system to a coordinated comprehensive system concerned with the maintenance of a maximum health condition and preventing, as well as dealing with illness. Such a reorientation coupled with a reorganization of the delivery system would incorporate the physician into an organizational network which coordinates his efforts with those of other medical and paramedical specialists. This would relieve the doctor of the need to spend his time performing tests and other functions which can be handled by specialists and technicians with lesser levels of training. It would also alter the existing concepts of needed physician/patient ratios thereby easing some of the upward pressure on the cost of medical care and partially relieving the shortage of fully trained physicians (Coe and Brehm, 1972, pp. 124–25).

Various health care delivery organization and financing mechanisms have been developed and tried in this country or have been proposed for adoption either following the experience in other countries or as a modification and extension of current techniques. Among these are some forms of national health insurance, as briefly commented on above, wider availability and use of the health maintenance organization approach, and increased use of physician extenders, nurse practitioners, and so on. Serious consideration should be given to the potential usefulness of these approaches, while still recognizing there are questions which need to be investigated relative to each of them.

National health insurance proposals of various forms have been submitted to the United States Congress over the last several years. Most of these proposals are purely mechanisms for financing the use of medical care services as they are currently delivered. That is, in general they advocate extending the principles involved in Medicare to the entire population. In essence, most of the national health insurance proposals would provide, in the form of a guarantee of payment, a financial overlay on the present health care delivery system.

It seems reasonable to anticipate that the United States will adopt some form of national health insurance as a mechanism for the financing of health care in the foreseeable future, given the variety of sources of support for such a move. At this juncture, it is highly probable that this program would include cost-sharing provisions in the form of deductibles and co–insurance.

If such a program is passed and implemented, it should be monitored for its impact on the availability, cost, and use of health services, including the effect on relative level of personal expenditures for these services. The different rates of use of different health services by men and women should be investigated more closely. This was noted specifically for older men and women under Medicare. Of particular concern would be an assessment of means to promote the increased use of ambulatory care services and the decreased use of in-patient facilities.

Pressures from the government and other third-party payors for cost control and accountability in medical institutions should result in some improvement in the use of hospital care, in terms of both average length of stay and rates of hospitalization. Since reduced rates of hospitalization often result in longer average lengths of stay, changes in both dimensions should be monitored closely and dealt with as interrelated but separable entities.

Concerns for cost control and appropriate use of the hospital as the most expensive facility should promote wider use of a variety of care levels, including skilled nursing facilities, out-patient ambulatory and day hospital services, and home health care, as means to shorten or avoid hospital stays. Research is needed on the efficiency and effectiveness of these alternate treatment modalities and levels in controlling costs of care. Analysis should be undertaken of the organizational factors, financing mechanisms, and decision-making control elements as they operate within and between provider units to influence general measures such as rates of use, average length of stay, patient cost, cost of an episode of care, and total population or area health care costs. Patterns of use of alternate treatment modalities and levels as these relate to the total costs of care, and the impact of changes and improvements in medical care technology on costs and efficiency in health care delivery should also be assessed.

Health maintenance organizations (HMOs) are prepaid group practice arrangements. Although there are many different mechanisms involved, the general intent is to provide coordinated, comprehensive health care services to members within an organizational and financing structure that offers incentives to the provider for delivering the care needed at the lowest possible cost. HMOs are potentially effective and cost-conscious approaches to the delivery of care. There are indications that they may be able to alter patterns of use of health care services on a long-term basis in favor of ambulatory care as a replacement for in-patient services, thereby reducing the total cost of care. Whether this is so because HMOs permit more rational planning or because they maintain a tight limit on the ratio of members to the in-patient hospital bed supply, the potential effect is the same (Brehm, 1978).

Fully packaged prepaid group plans that own and operate their own hospitals, skilled nursing facilities, and so on, could be an effective device for providing coordinated, comprehensive care. Research will be needed to establish the value of these plans to contain costs and hold down utilization, particularly of the more expensive in-patient facilities, without reducing the quality of care. The impact on cost and use of different organizational patterns and physician reimbursement mechanisms both within and outside of such HMOs should be evaluated.

Physician extenders and nurse practitioners are two titles in use to identify personnel who, as less highly paid, less highly trained persons, can substitute for direct physician services in situations not requiring a physician's level of knowledge and skill, thereby freeing the physician for more complicated tasks.

Additional research must be undertaken on the most effective means to utilize these personnel so as to increase the overall quality of care while stabilizing the demand for physician services and the costs of such care. Additional problems still remain in institutionalizing the use of such personnel within the delivery system. More research is needed on such problems as mechanisms for financing and payment, the requirements for licensure and the permissible functions for such persons as they differ from state to state, malpractice insurance complications, and general acceptance by both physicians and patients of such staff so as to promote the smoothest transition to maximum use.

These mechanisms deal with the interrelated problem areas of manpower, facilities, and services at appropriate levels of care, and the cost and financing of such care. The provision of coordinated, comprehensive care requires sound planning and assessment of alternate delivery mechanisms. There is no shortage of ideas on how to improve the organization and financing of health care delivery. However, there are limitations in authority to direct the implementation of various delivery approaches or to coordinate or control the health care delivery system. Additionally, we need an expanded base of knowledge about which mechanisms and organizational combinations will most effectively accomplish the dual purpose of providing high quality medical care without waste of resources or intolerably high costs.

Elements of a National Health Policy

There are, of course, many ways in which the specifics of a health care *program* could be defined. Examples of some of these variations are found in the different legislative proposals now before Congress, but it is neither necessary nor useful to review these here. Rather, it is more appropriate to outline some general guides for a *policy* based on experiences with Medicare. In so doing, it is assumed that the right to good health will continue to be supported and that it will be politically more feasible to fashion a system by integration of already existing public and private resources than to maintain the status quo. Some key elements in a national policy might include the following:

Universal coverage: A national program should be truly national in scope and include all members of the population, for whom there should be equal benefits. Payment mechanisms could include both public and private third-party intermediaries, but some form of prepayment (with subsidization for the poor) should replace the current fee-for-service payment system. Furthermore, the current concepts of deductibles and co-insurance should be discontinued. With Medicare, their function to deter "unnecessary" utilization was more than offset by preventing some elderly from obtaining needed services, and they may well have affected the choice of care mechanism in the direction of those forms requiring the smallest relative amount of out-of-pocket expenditure.

Comprehensive care: Services included in the program must extend to all levels of care—primary, secondary, and tertiary. One of the failures of Medicare was to impose the concept of "spell of illness" on the use of inpatient acute and intermediate-care facilities when they were being used for chronic diseases, and to exclude some ambulatory and home-based services altogether. A plan must be devised for facilitating movement of patients from one level and source of care to another more appropriate level. In this respect, there should be a greater emphasis on preventive social and health services and a de-emphasis on institutionally based care.

Health personnel management: Two main issues of concern are the disproportionate numbers of specialists among health professionals and their maldistribution in the population. The first can be affected especially for physicians by eliminating fee-for-services payments and by increasing financial support for training programs in primary care. Distribution of personnel can be influenced by increased subsidization of students during training in return for assigned tours of duty in underserved areas. Both of these techniques are being used already, but need to be expanded. Another personnel dimension is better integration of health professionals into teams and increased use of allied health personnel in programs of expanded primary care services.

Regulation: One of the major failures of the current Medicare program was its lack of influence on the provision of services, other than payment for them. Clearly, a more forceful and more broadly based community group is needed to regulate the distribution of resources and compel an integration of heretofore independent and competitive facilities and services. This calls for participation of a broader range of professionals and citizens' groups than is currently the case.

Health education: All of the foregoing is based on the assumption of an informed public. Experience to date suggests this is an untenable assumption. Thus, policy should require that a means be developed to educate the public in appropriate use of an integrated and comprehensive health care system. In fact, some special attention must be given to training health *professionals,* to use and work in such a system.

One approach that should be given serious and unemotional consideration is the instituting of a national program involving direct control over the system for delivery of health care services, as exists in various other countries. Unquestionably, a proposal for such an approach would face political opposition, particularly from organized medicine but also from various other medical care groups. However, in view of the problems related to Medicare, a program involving control over the delivery system must be seen as a viable alternative to or modification of extending the Medicare approach to the entire population under some form of national health insurance.

Direct public control over the medical care delivery system could be instituted to operate, in at least a limited sphere of activity, on two levels. Responsibility for overall policy would be centralized and would include resource development planning, personnel training, resource allocation among areas, and establishment of guidelines for coordinated use of the various levels of health care. This centralized policy activity would facilitate the implementation of knowledge gained through studies of incentives to control cost, optional organizational arrangements, interrelationships among facilities and levels of care, and the use of special personnel such as physician extenders and nurse practitioners (Brehm, 1978).

Coordinating the various providers of medical care should be done at the regional or local level. As discussed, the direct delivery of care is performed at the local level. Coordination could control the unwarranted duplication and overlap of services and facilities among units and the inappropriate use of various levels of care. Assuring that needed care modalities are available and accessible can also be most effectively done at the regional or local level.

Such controls can probably be implemented most reasonably by incorporating them within the structure of whatever national health insurance program is adopted in the United States. Any such program adopted probably will not have a meaningful level of direct system control in its original form. These controls would have to be added later as experience under the program reaffirmed that a system that guaranteed payment but exercised no direct control over the delivery system could not accomplish its purposes, with or without cost containment.

Such a program would have the explicit intent of removing the financial barriers to health care through guaranteed payment for care received; the implicit intent would be to promote the availability of care appropriate to the health needs of the population (Brehm, 1978).

It was more than 50 years from the first mention of government-sponsored, compulsory health insurance to the passage of Medicare. The lessons of these first years of Medicare have been thoroughly explored. Let us hope that the necessary changes to policy or program can be made more expeditiously.

BIBLIOGRAPHY

Anderson, O. W. *Health care: Can there be equity?* New York: Wiley, 1972.

Bodenheimer, T. S. The hoax of national health insurance. *American Journal of Public Health*, October 1972, *62*; 1325–1327.

Braybrooke, D., & Lindholm, C. E., *A strategy of decision* (Policy evaluation as a social process). Glencoe, Ill.: The Free Press, 1963.

Brehm, H. P. The future of U.S. health care delivery for the elderly. In *Aging and income*, edited by B. R. Herzog, chap. 7. New York: Human Sciences Press, 1978.

Brown, J. D. *An American philosophy of social security: Evaluation and issues.* Princeton, N. J.: Princeton University Press, 1972.

Chapman, C. B., & Talmadge, J. M. Evolution of the right to health concept in the United States. *Humanistic perspectives in medical ethics*, edited by M. B. Visscher. Buffalo, N.Y.: Prometheus Books, 1972, pp. 72–134.

Clarke, H. *Social Legislation*, 2d ed. New York: Appleton-Century-Crofts, 1957.

Coe, R. M. Assessment of preventive health care practices for the aged. *Gerontologist*, Autumn 1973, *13*, 345–358.

Coe, R. M. *Sociology of medicine*, 2d ed. New York: McGraw Hill, 1978.

Coe, R. M., and Asociates *Medicare report: Evaluation of the provision and utilization of community health resources.* Kansas City: Institute for Community Studies, 1970.

Coe, R. M., & Brehm, H. P. *Preventive health care for adults.* New Haven: College and University Press Services, 1972.

Coe, R. M., Brehm, H. P., & Peterson, W. A. Impact of medicine on the organization of community health resources. *Milbank Memorial Fund Quarterly Health and Society*, Summer 1974, *52*, 231–264.

Coe, R. M., Peterson, W. A., Sigler, J., Stroker, M., & Edgerton, J. *Impact of Medicare in selected communities.* Institute for Community Studies, Kansas City, Mo., Final Report SSA Contract No. 71–3400, April 1973.

Coe, R. M., & Sigler, J. Physicians' perspectives on the impact of Medicare. *Medical Care*, January–February 1970, *8*, 26–34.

Colombotos, J. Physician attitudes towards Medicare. *Medical Care*, July–August 1968, *6*, 320–331.

Colombotos, J. Physicians and Medicare: A before-after study of the effects of legislation on attitudes. *American Sociological Review*, June 1969, *34*, 318–334.

Committee for National Health Insurance. *Month Report 2*, December 1975, p. 2.

Congressional Record. Cviii, March 5, 1962, pp. 3112–3113.

Crawford, R. You are dangerous to your health: The ideology and politics of victim blaming. *International Journal of Health Services*, 1977, *7*, No. 4, 663–680.

Davis, K. Equal treatment and unequal benefits: The Medicare program. *Milbank Memorial Fund Quarterly*, 1975, *53* (4), 449–488.

Dexter, L. A. *Tyranny of schooling; An inquiry into the problem of stupidity.* New York: Basic Books, 1964.

137

Epstein, L. A., & Murray, J. H. *The aged population of the United States: The 1963 Social Security survey of the aged.* Social Security Administration, Research Report 19. Washington, D.C., 1967.

Feder, J. M. Medicare implementation and the policy process. *Journal of Health Politics, Policy and Law,* Summer 1977, *2,* 173–189.

Feingold, E. *Medicare: Policy and politics.* San Francisco: Chandler, 1966.

Flexner, J. T. *Doctors on horseback.* New York: Dover, 1968.

Freidson, E. *Profession of medicine: A study of the sociology of applied knowledge.* New York: Dodd, Mead and Co., 1972.

Gibson, R. M., & Mueller, M. S. National health expenditure highlights, fiscal year 1976. *Research and Statistics Note,* Note No. 27, December 22, 1976. Social Security Administration, Office of Research and Statistics.

Gordon, G., Anderson, O. W., Brehm, H. P., & Marquis, S. *Disease, the individual and society.* New Haven: College and University Press, 1968.

Gornick, M. Ten years of Medicare: Impact on the covered population. *Social Security Bulletin,* July 1976, *39,* 3–21.

Harris, R. Annals of Legislation. *New Yorker Magazine,* July 2, 9, 16, and 23, 1966.

Harris, R. *A sacred trust.* Baltimore: Pelican, 1969.

Howards, I., Brehm, H. P., & Nagi, S. Z. *Disability: From social problem to federal program.* New York: Praeger, 1980.

Jonsen, A. R. Principles for an ethics of health services. In *Social policy, social ethics and the aging society,* edited by B. L. Neugarten and R. J. Havighurst. Washington, D.C.: U.S. Government Printing Office, 1976.

Knowles, J. Getting better and feeling worse. *Daedalus, 1977.*

Larson, R. Thirty years of research on the subjective well-being of older Americans. *Journal of Gerontology,* 1978, *33,* 109–125.

Longest, B. B., Jr. The U.S. health care system. In *Health, illness, and medicine, a reader in medical sociology,* edited by G. L. Albrecht and P. C. Higgins, chap. 22. Chicago: Rand McNally College Publishing Co., 1979.

MacColl, W. A. *Group practice and prepayment of medical care.* Washington, D.C.: Public Affairs Press, 1966.

McKeown, T. Planning for geriatric services in Britain. *Gerontologist,* June 1964, 4, 18–24.

Myers, R. J. *Medicare.* New York: Irwin, 1970.

Munan, L., Vobecky, J., & Kelly, A. Population health care practices: An epidemiologic study of the immediate effects of a universal health insurance plan. *International Journal of Health Services,* 1974, *4,* 285–295.

National Center for Health Statistics. *Health insurance,* Series 10, No. 16. Washington, D.C.: National Center for Health Statistics, 1965a.

National Center for Health Statistics. *Volume of physician visits,* Series 10, No. 18. Washington, D.C.: National Center for Health Statistics, 1965b.

National Center for Health Statistics. *Characteristics of residents in institutions for the aged and chronically ill, U.S.—April–June 1963,* Series 12, No. 2. Washington, D.C.: National Center for Health Statistics, 1965c.

National Center for Health Statistics. *Utilization of short stay hospitals,* Series 13, No. 2. Washington, D.C.: National Center for Health Statistics, 1965d.

National Center for Health Statistics. *Characteristics of residents in nursing and personal care homes, U.S.—June–August 1969*, Series 12, No. 19. Washington, D.C.: National Center for Health Statistics, 1973.

National Center for Health Statistics. Current estimates from the health interview survey, 1968. Series 10, No. 60. Washington, D.C.: National Center for Health Statistics, 1970.

National Center for Health Statistics. *Utilization of nursing homes, U.S.:—August 1973–April 1974*, Series 13, No. 28. Washington, D.C.: National Center for Health Statistics, 1977.

National Center for Health Statistics. *Physician visits*, Series 10, No. 97. Washington, D.C.: National Center for Health Statistics, 1975.

National Center for Health Statistics. *Physician visits*, Series 10, No. 126. Washington, D.C.: National Center for Health Statistics, 1978.

National Center for Health Statistics. *Physician visits*, Series 10, No. 128. Washington, D.C.: National Center for Health Statistics, 1979.

Perkins, F. *The roots of Social Security*. Printed remarks of October 23, 1962, address to a general staff meeting of the Social Security Administration in Baltimore, Maryland. U.S. Department of Health, Education, and Welfare, Social Security Administration, August 1963, EP17, Baltimore, Maryland.

Ruther, M. Equal treatment and unequal benefits: A re-examination of the use of Medicare services by race, 1967–1976. Paper presented American Public Health Association Annual Meeting, November 6, 1979.

Ryan, W. *Blaming the victim*, rev. ed. New York: Vintage, 1976.

Sanders, D. S. *The impact of reform movements on social policy change: The case of social insurance*. Fairlawn, N.J.: R. E. Burdick, 1973.

Shanas, E. Social myth as hypothesis: The case of family relations of old people. *Gerontologist*, February 1979, *19*, 3–9.

Shanas, E. & Maddox, G. L. Aging, health and the organization of health resources. In, *Handbook of aging and the social sciences*, edited by R H. Binstock and E. Shanas. New York: Van Nostrand, 1976.

Siegel, J. S. Prospective trends in the size and structure of the elderly population; Impact of mortality trends and some implications. *Current Population Reports*, January 1979, Series P–23, No. 78.

Shonick, W. The public hospital and its local ecology in the United States. *International Journal of Health Services*, 1979, 9, 359–396.

Social Security Handbook, 6th ed. U.S. Department of Health, Education, and Welfare, Social Security Administration, HEW Publication No. (SSA) 77–10135, Washington, D.C., July 1978.

Stevens, R., & Stevens, R. *Welfare medicine in America: a case study of Medicaid*. New York: Free Press, 1974.

Tyler, P. (ed.) *Social welfare in the United States*. The Reference Shelf, Vol. 27, No. 3. New York: H. W. Wilson, 1955.

U.S. Congress, Senate, Committee on Finance. *The Social Security Act and related laws (as amended through December 31, 1976)*. 94th Cong., 2d sess. Washington, D.C.: U.S. Government Printing Office, 1976.

U.S. Department of Commerce, Bureau of the Census. *Statistical abstract of the*

United States, 1967. Washington, D.C.: U.S. Government Printing Office, 1967.

U.S. Department of Commerce, Bureau of the Census. *Statistical abstract of the United States, 1975.* Washington, D.C.: U.S. Government Printing Office, 1975.

U.S. Department of Health, Education, and Welfare. *Medicare 1967*, Section 1.2, Summary. Social Security Administration, Office of Research and Statistics.

U.S. Department of Health, Education, and Welfare. *Compendium of national health expenditure data*, DHEW Pub. No. (SSA76-11927). Washington, D.C.: U.S. Department of Health, Education, and Welfare, 1976(a).

U.S. Department of Health, Education and Welfare. *Medicare, fiscal years 1969-1973.* Selected state data. DHEW Pub. No. (SSA76-11711). Washington, D.C.: Social Security Administration, 1976. (b)

U.S. Department of Health, Education, and Welfare. *Medicare, 1975-76*, Section 1.2, Summary. Health Care Financing Administration, Office of Policy, Planning and Research.

Weil, P. Comparative costs to the Medicare program of seven prepaid group practices and controls. *Health and Society*, Summer 1976, *54*, 339-365.

West, H. Five years of Medicare—A statistical review. *Social Security Bulletin*, 1971, *34* (12), 17-27.

Your Medicare Handbook. U.S. Department of Health, Education and Welfare, Social Security Administration, DHEW Publication No. (SSA) 76-10050, January 1976.

INDEX

ABOUT THE AUTHORS

HENRY P. BREHM is Adjunct Associate Professor of Sociology at the University of Maryland Baltimore County. He has been affiliated with the University since 1969.

Dr. Brehm has authored and co-authored a series of journal articles and other presentations in the area of sociology. He also is a co-author on the following books: *Disease, the Individual, and Society; Preventive Health Care for Adults;* and, *Disability, From Social Problem to Federal Program.*

Dr. Brehm holds a B.A. and M.A. from New York University and a Ph.D. from the University of Maryland College Park.

RODNEY M. COE, Ph.D., is Professor of Community Medicine, Saint Louis University School of Medicine, St. Louis, Missouri. He received the Ph.D. in Sociology from Washington University in 1962. From 1963 to 1973 he was director of the Medical Care Research Center in Saint Louis. In addition to articles in professional journals, Dr. Coe is author of *Sociology of Medicine* (1978), editor of *Planned Change in the Hospital* (1970), and co-author with M. Pepper of *Community Medicine: Some New Perspectives* (1978), and with Henry Brehm, *Preventive Care for Adults* (1972).